Health Cooperation with Russia

Health Cooperation with Russia

An Example of Engagement that Really Worked

Edward J. Burger Jr.
M.D., Sc.D., MACP

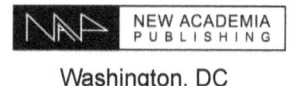

Washington, DC

Copyright © 2017 by Edward J. Burger Jr.

New Academia Publishing, 2017

All rights reserved. No part of this book may be reproduced or transmitted in any form or by any means, electronic or mechanical, including photocopying, recording, or by any information storage and retrieval system.

Printed in the United States of America

Library of Congress Control Number: 2017943304
ISBN 978-0-9986433-3-5 paperback (alk. paper)

Contents

Acknowledgements	iv
Preface	v
Chapter 1. A Brief History of the Russian and Soviet Health Care System	1
Chapter 2. The State of Affairs in the Early 1990s	7
Chapter 3. The Gestation Period 1995-1997	15
Chapter 4. The Program	25
Chapter 5. The Results: What the Program Accomplished	49
Chapter 6. Health: An Instrument of Engagement	63
Epilogue	69
Notes	72
About the Author	79
Index	81

Acknowledgements

I want to acknowledge the essential contribution made to the success of this program by my colleagues, Richard Farmer, MD, and Harvey Sloane, MD.

Preface

As this review is being written, twenty-five years have past since the implosion of the Soviet Union. Over that span, U.S.-Russian relations have followed an uneven path, marked by extreme highs and extreme lows. Angela Stent, in her book The Limits of Partnerships, counts four identifiable, explicit efforts at cooperation. Some of these were initiated by the United States, and some originated with the Russian Federation. All of these attempts eventually faltered. The depth of the current relationship between the two countries has been variously termed a "nadir" or one that is so troubled as to need "life support."

The political tensions that mark U.S.-Russian relations have raised the strategic choice of isolation from or cooperation with Russia. As one with direct involvement in U.S.-Russian relations over the course of more than forty years, this author comes down squarely in favor of taking advantage of cooperative opportunities.

The Eurasian Medical Education Program of the American College of Physicians was originally conceived simply as an effort to share scientific and clinical medical experience with members of the Russian medical profession. The background was seventy years of isolation of the Russian medical profession from western medicine. The pattern chosen for this sharing was a practice observed around the world in medicine, termed continuing medical education. Physician exchanges with Russian regional academic medical centers were the vehicle. Over the seventeen years of the program, we interacted with well in excess of ten thousand Russian practitioners. A key element in the success of the program was a high level of professional contribution on both sides. The interchanges were arranged to provide exposure of the visiting American medical experts to Russian experience and knowledge as well.

A nominal goal of the Eurasian Medical Education Program was the enhancement of the technical capacity of Russian physicians to manage serious disease. But the program demonstrated an additional contribution at least as important as the original one - that health and medicine are effective instruments of engagement. Unlike other sectors, medicine is politically neutral. By contrast, rule of law, for example, carries with it substantial political overtones. Thus, while the seventeen-year period of the Eurasian Medical Education Program in Russia was marked by nearly constant political turmoil, the program was entirely untouched by that politically tumultuous environment. A 2012 declaration by the Russian government forbade programs supported by the U.S. Agency for International Development because of the emphasis of those programs on human rights, democracy promotion, and open support for opposition political parties. Support for cooperation in the medical sector was preserved. In fact, the Eurasian Medical Education Program and its leadership were afforded professional recognition at the highest level of the medical and scientific establishment.

1

A Brief History of the Russian and Soviet Health Care System

In order to appreciate the state of medicine that we found in the early 1990s, it is useful to take account of what preceded that period, going as far back as the middle of the nineteenth century. Russian medicine had undergone a series of substantial changes in organization and support, all reflective of dynamic changes in political and governmental goals and the particular position of medicine in serving those goals.

Two notable trends are apparent throughout this period, although the weight and direction given to them varied. One was the emphasis given to prevention of disease—motivated by the specter of typhus and other infectious processes. The other was the need felt by political leaders to reach the widely dispersed population in the vast country.[1] This was illustrated at various times by the changing view at the top of the administration to distribute political power or, alternatively to centrally control it. This move recognized the need to accommodate the health needs of this broadly distributed rural population. It includes the establishment of a "stationing system"—a network of medical stations, dispensaries, and hospitals.

Roughly a decade later in 1864, Emperor Alexander II, recognizing the need for administrative reform, established the zemtsvo system of governance. This was a substantial redistribution of political power to the periphery through a delegation to zemtsvo (district) governing units throughout the country. Jurisdiction of health, alongside education, in Russia reached its full flowering under the zemtsvo system.[2]

Zemtsvo medicine was the first attempt to give organized medical services to the rural population. (Anton Chekov was a zemtsvo physician.) The zemtsvo system created a network of medical stations throughout the country. Medicine and its practitioners came to be seen as professionals and the system as a public utility.[3] Further, whereas many among the physician community had been of foreign origin, after the middle of the nineteenth century, the leading medical scientists were Russian.[4]

The zemtsvo system remained in place until the Bolshevik revolution of 1917. The revolution eventually brought major changes to the role and position of physicians. Doctors offered their services to the new regime but effectively were rejected as elitist and feared politically active. Further and ironically, as upholders of the announced ethic of universal care, the new regime insisted on a system of hierarchical class treatment. Physicians were made employees of the state and were remunerated at the rate of 70% of the average industrial wage.[5]

Within five days following the Bolshevik revolution, the new regime announced a concept of social insurance. Medical care was to be universally available and free. All health activities were to be directed by a central authority. Health care was to be planned on a large scale. The cost burden for this sector was to be placed on employers and considered as a cost of production.

While the Russian physician in 1917, at the beginning of the revolution, resembled members of the profession elsewhere in the world, the new Soviet leadership was suspicious of the medical profession but did not at first mount a frontal assault on it. The Bolsheviks wanted a benevolent neutrality or at least collaboration. While these intentions were announced, they were not realized for another five years, pending the resolution of social turmoil and a civil war. But change did come.

The new regime moved to emphasize social factors as the principal contributors to disease. Clinical medicine was downgraded in importance. Public health and personal medical care were deemed to be state responsibilities. A semiautonomous medical profession and organized professional medical societies were incompatible with the new socialist goals. Importantly, this resulted in the loss of elements of professionalism that had traditionally shaped the behavior of the medical profession. Medical teaching institutions were separated from the general university system. The Academy of Medical Sciences was separated from the Soviet Academy of Sciences. There ensued a prolonged period of restrictions on professional activities such as meetings, professional publications, and travel.

Beginning in the 1930s, the Stalin regime gave large political weight to industrialization and collective agriculture. Emphasis was on production and industrial output. Medicine became an instrument in behalf of production. That year saw the creation of the All-Union Commissariat of Health, devoted to further centralization of planning and control, resulting in an enormous increase in professional and physical resources for health. As a result, the Soviet Union could claim twice the number of physicians per capita than the United States and three times the number of hospital beds.[6] This had a marked effect on the management of disease. Patients were "processed" rather than treated. Soviet citizens were much more likely to be admitted to hospital than their western counterparts. If admitted, Soviet patients remained in hospital for long periods of time.

Financial support for the medical care system came from the state budget. Throughout the Soviet period, payments to physicians were kept very low. This contributed to a pattern of out-of-pocket spending by patients and their families ("envelope-passing medicine"), which became established as a necessary path to adequate care. Financial support for the medical care system eventually fell into a decline. The percentage of Soviet gross domestic product (GDP) officially allocated to the health care system between 1955 and 1977 decreased more than 20%.[7] As Mark Field observed, medicine in the Soviet Union must be understood against a "background of scarcities, the bureaucracy, the officiousness of state employees, the absurdities of formal rules and the inequities from top to bottom."[8]

As the general economic decline worsened in the 1980s, the decline of the social security system was paralleled by a general disintegration of the system of medical care. By the beginning of the 1990s, the economy was in free fall as a result of a precipitous decline in production and a lack of efficient markets and industrial exchange. The nation was able to fund only 60% of health care in

Russia.[9] The parallel deterioration of the economy and the health system led to a decline in indices of health, beginning in the 1970s By 1993, the portion of the government budget devoted to health had declined to 3.2%.[10] A result was a steady deterioration in the state of health.

Toward the end of the nineteenth century, life expectancy at birth in Russia fell short of the comparable record in western Europe. For example, during the period 1896 to 1897, life expectancy in Russia was thirty-two years compared to forty-seven years in France and the United States.[11] By 1938 to 1939, Soviet life expectancy had reached forty-three years, but the gap between the Soviet experience and that in France or the United States had widened further.

Following World War II, life expectancy in the Soviet Union rose so rapidly that the gap with western Europe was dramatically reduced. By 1965, male life expectancy in the Soviet Union, which had reached 64.3 years, lagged behind that in western Europe by only a couple of years. The gap between the U.S. experience and that of the Soviet Union at this time was only a bit over two years.[12]

By the latter part of the 1960s, progress in life expectancy had slowed. Life expectancy in the Soviet Union and that in western Europe and the U.S. began to move in opposite directions, with stagnation or even deterioration in the case of the Soviet Union. The principal contributors to premature or excess mortality were cardiovascular and cerebrovascular disease and causes of trauma. Adult premature mortality showed a nearly consistent decline from 1965 onward and continued over the next three decades. A temporary, two-year pause occurred in 1988 with the issuance of a resolution for "actions against drunkenness and alcoholism."[13] The campaign ended with the collapse of the political and economic structure of the Soviet Union in the period 1989 to 1991, and the deterioration of health indices resumed.

Excess male mortality was most striking, leading to a male/female life expectancy gap of nearly 14 years.[14] Overwhelmingly, the major contributors to this pattern were cardiovascular disease and consequences of trauma and violence. The contribution of cardiovascular and cerebrovascular disease far exceeded all of the mortality from infectious disease.

As premature mortality in Russia increased, it was accompanied by decreased fertility. The consequence of these two was a dramatic demographic decline. In the first nine months of 1993, Moscow saw two and one-half times as many deaths as births.[15] This negative "natural population increase" was a net yearly loss of four hundred thousand to six hundred thousand individuals per year net of any in-migration, or a loss of 0.6% of the population. Further, the pattern of excess mortality was most prominent among the sectors mostly thought of as potentially most productive—young and middle-aged males (see table 1). Russian population decline was without precedent outside of wartime and other disasters with consequent important implications for economic development.

Table 1. Life expectancy at birth, men and women in Russia, 1979–1997

Year	Men	Women	Differential (in years, female by male)
1979–80	61.5	73.0	11.5
1980–81	61.5	73.1	11.6
1981–82	62.0	73.5	11.5
1982–83	62.3	73.6	11.3
1983–84	62.0	73.3	11.3
1984–85	62.3	73.3	11.0
1985–86	63.8	74.0	10.2
1986–87	64.9	74.6	9.7
1988	64.8	74.4	9.6
1989	64.2	74.5	10.3
1990	63.8	74.3	10.5
1991	63.5	74.3	10.8
1992	62.0	73.8	11.8
1993	58.9	71.9	13.0
1994	57.6	71.2	13.6
1995	58.3	71.7	13.4
1996	59.8	72.5	12.7
1997	60.8	72.9	12.1

Source: *Russia's Torn Safety Nets: Health and Social Welfare During the Transition*, ed. Mark G. Field and Judyth L. Twigg (New York: St. Martin's Press, 2000).

2

The State of Affairs in the Early 1990s

The sudden implosion of the Soviet Union caught many by surprise. Appropriate western response was uncertain and became the subject of debate lasting several years in the 1990s. Several proposals were made to provide Marshall Plan-type funding to assist the Russian Federation over an anticipated difficult transition. One of the proposals of the time was made in 1992 by the Harvard economist Jeffrey Sachs. Sachs noted that Russia had inherited the external debt of the Soviet Union. He reasoned that, because the G-7 countries had failed to develop a coherent strategy to support economic reforms in Russia, the reform effort would be weakened, resulting in adverse consequences to multiple parties. He predicted an acute balance-of-payments crisis and an acute fiscal crisis, threatening hyperinflation made worse by the debts inherited from the Soviet Union. He pointed to the inevitable shocks that would accompany the transition to a democratic society and a market-based economy.

His proposal was for a $27 billion fund to be derived from bilateral sources and from international financial institutions.[1] Most important for this discussion, roughly a third of these monies were to have been devoted to a "social fund" to pay for health care and other social costs to tide over the nation during the difficult transition.[2] Others joined this argument, urging western support for stabilization of the ruble.[3] Sachs, in the end, was not persuasive; his proposals to the G-7 were not adopted and were even savagely attacked in some academic quarters.[4]

Independent of these proposals but more or less concurrently, there occurred much discussion of the merits of other large-scale initiatives for Russia.[5] In November 1992, the World Bank briefly considered a "Marshall Plan type technical assistance program for the former Soviet Union." The accompanying memorandum proposed that "...the political timing is propitious for a massive, post-Cold War effort similar in spirit to the original postwar program."[6]

Most of these proposals were rejected, not on the basis of need or merit, but with the argument that, unlike postwar Europe, Russia did not possess the banking, legal, and other institutions or experience to use these funds effectively.[7] Ironically, these same critics admitted that "The Marshall Plan [had been] a testing ground for the conversion of Germany from enemy into partner" and "History tells us that vindictive policies breed revolution while incorporation provides greater security than the Maginot Line."[8]

Early U.S. Initiatives

Some of the earliest health and social assistance programs for Russia, following dissolution of the Soviet system, were humanitarian and food assistance projects and donation of decommissioned military hospital equipment in 1992 and 1993. A more significant initiative began in 1992 when Secretary of State James Baker convened the Washington Coordinating Conference on Assistance to the New Independent States. The purpose was to determine appropriate humanitarian assistance for the former Soviet states. One of the products of this inquiry was an initiative known as the Medical Working Group: Experts Delegation to the Newly Independent States. This was a delegation of thirty health care professionals from thirteen countries who visited medical institutions and public health authorities in ten of the former Soviet republics. (One of the numerous ironies associated with this mission was that the vehicle that transported the delegates from country to country was a NATO airplane.) The terms of reference for this mission were forward looking and included a spirit both of humanitarian assistance and provision of longer-term professional cooperation. Goals included coordination of the provision of medicines and medical supplies, and a search for opportunities for private sector involvement and encouragement of cooperative professional partnerships with U.S. medical institutions.

In Russia, the delegates foresaw a loosening of the authority of the centralized federal ministries of health, a further decline in the financial resources available to the health care system, and a growing number of citizens without access to care.[9] The delegates recognized the extensive delivery system already in place. But because of lack of financing, Russia was experiencing an exodus of scientists and a deterioration of the elements of basic social services. They acknowledged that humanitarian assistance can have an "anesthetizing effect" on recipients. Most important, at every stop the delegates met with an admonition from the Russian hosts to diminish donor humanitarian assistance instead "help us help ourselves."[10]

In the wake of the Medical Working Group's mission, the United States Agency for International Development (USAID) put in place a highly meritorious initiative known initially as the Hospital Partnership Program. This was a linkage with professional exchanges among twenty-six American hospitals and twenty-six counterpart institutions in the former Soviet republics. The majority of the linkages and exchanges were built around clinical subjects corresponding to the major burdens of disease for Russians — notably cardiovascular disease, tuberculosis, obstetrics and gynecology, pediatrics. The program, which eventually became known as the American International Health Alliance, changed its character with time and moved away from its original focus of professional, clinical medical exchanges. Over the next few years USAID instituted some additional initiatives, including the Rational Pharmaceutical Project, and provided support for programs that addressed tuberculosis in five of Russia's political regions.

Alongside these successful efforts, USAID was responsible for what can only be called some misguided adventures. The most prominent of these, the Health Reform Project, was started in 1993, had as its commission the remaking of health care organization and financing in five regions of the former Soviet Union. The focus was entirely on economics and organization. Yet results, in terms of betterment of health, were expected to be realized in political time.[11] USAID had planned to spend $75 million on this program. Because its overall goal and its administration were deeply flawed, it was prematurely closed down after an expenditure of only $44 million.[12]

Early International Efforts

In the first few years of the 1990s, a large number of countries and international institutions undertook a similar review of needs and opportunities in te former Soviet republics. For example, the World Bank, suddenly finding itself challenged by a rash of fifteen new members (Russia and the other new members of the Commonwealth of Independent States), mounted an exercise to determine a proper role for health and social welfare.

The World Bank scrambled to assemble country-centered programs for each of the new independent states. As noted above, there was an early consideration of a Marshall Plan type of initiative for the former Soviet Union, which ultimately did not materialize.in the early 1990s, the World Bank took an interest in the process, which led to the replacement of state funding for medical care in Russia by an obligatory insurance program.[13] For a few years, the World Bank fostered a Medical Equipment Project in Russia. In 1998 the president of the World Bank announced an accelerated loan program of $150 million for tuberculosis and HIV/AIDS for Russia.

There were other modest initiatives—bilateral programs paid for by the Technical Aid to the Commonwealth of Independent States (TACIS) of the European Union; Department for International Development (DIFID) of the United Kingdom and Scandinavian, Canadian, and German governments. In many of these cases, tuberculosis was the focus of interest.

The International Monetary Fund (IMF) calculated that Russia alone would require at least $20 billion in outside assistance to meet its foreign exchange needs in both 1992 and 1993. As they put together programs of assistance in those years, the G-7 governments anticipated that the bulk of the financing would come from the international financial institutions—the IMF, World Bank, and European Development Bank. As was later noted in a report from the Congressional Research Office, both the IMF and World Bank promised much less than had been anticipated.[14] In April 1992, the G-7 proposed $10.5 billion in multilateral assistance for Russia, including a $6 billion ruble stabilization fund. In the end, only $1.6 billion was offered.[15] An irony of this story is that, from the beginning, the IMF recognized the vital importance of supporting the social structure of Russia during the transition.[16]

Decline in Support for Russia

What of private, philanthropic foundations—the so-called independent sector? When the Soviet Union collapsed, private foundation support for area studies and arms control studies fell away dramatically. The job was completed, these institutions reasoned. To their credit, some prominent foundations raised attention to ill health in Russia and the consequent implications for security of a falling population.[17] However, only two major foundations supported operational programs for health assistance in the Russian Federation—the Soros Foundation and the Bill and Melinda Gates Foundation. Unfortunately, support from this quarter was short-lived.

In the early 1990s, there was strong Congressional support for assistance for Russia. Congress enacted the Freedom Support Act in 1992 and made provision for the office of Coordinator in the State Department, to be responsible for strategic planning for the orderly and rational provision of that assistance. The office was also to provide assistance in the social and health sectors but that was never adequately funded. As one reviewer noted, "Although the idea of providing a social safety net was supported by a number of prominent analysts...the United States never considered it as something it could do alone—it would require massive sums."[18]

By 1995, there were clear signs that the Congressional consensus for support for Russia had begun to fall apart. The foreign assistance budget for Russia, $1.3 billion in 1994, dropped to $168 million in 1996. Critical questions were raised about the effectiveness of those expenditures, about the excessive use of consultants and large contractors, and about the focus of the assistance. These criticisms combined with frank savaging of the notion that fostering a strong Russia was even desirable.[19] It was against this U.S. policy response to an increasing death rate and declining population that the Eurasian Medical Education Program was born.

Origins of the Eurasian Medical Education Program

The concept of the Eurasian Medical Education Program originated with two individuals -- the author and a colleague, Dr. Richard Farmer. Both of us were faculty members of the Georgetown University Medical Center. Dr. Farmer had served for a period as a medical scientist for USAID and was one of the leaders of the Medical Working Group delegation to Russia. I had dealt with Soviet matters earlier in the White House Office of the President's Science Adviser. In the early 1970s, the U.S. Government, on the initiative of the Science Advisor, developed a series of cooperative research programs with the USSR in health, science, and the environment, and I helped bring these about.

The original concept for the Eurasian Medical Education Program emerged from exploration of a single question: What initiative could be developed that promised to make a real contribution to the health challenge in Russia? The dimensions of the challenge included a country of enormous size (eleven time zones), a heavily overbuilt health care system, a national expenditure of approximately only 4% of GNP, and diminished indices of health. In considering answers to the question, the factor that stood out above all was the seventy-year isolation of the medical profession from western medicine and medical science. The rules of the Soviet period had not permitted physicians to interact with the rest of the professional world. This fact immediately pointed to an opportunity for a program designed to share knowledge, experience, and skills with colleagues. The recognized institutional vehicle for this activity around the world is known as Continuing Medical Education. Typically, physicians everywhere are obliged to return periodically to educational sessions to experience what new science has come to the profession and what are considered contemporary standards of care in managing disease.

Continuing postgraduate medical education was adopted as the basic concept for what became the Eurasian Medical Education Program. The vehicle for the program would be professional physician exchanges involving physicians trained in internal medicine and its subspecialties. They would spend one to two weeks in academic medical centers in Russia in lectures, seminars, and clinical teaching rounds with patients.

In 1996, Dr. Farmer and I held a series of discussions with the leadership of the American Medical Association (AMA) to explore a possible partnership arrangement. After a six-month period of deliberation, the AMA decided to decline cooperation, citing a beleaguered medical profession in the U.S. with too many intrinsic problems and with the summary excuse, "why help the evil empire?"

More fruitful discussions were held with the leadership of the American College of Physicians (ACP), a long-standing(since 1915) professional organization of 130,000 internal medicine physicians. The principal activity of the ACP is postgraduate physician education. The ACP had in place a number professional ties with medical societies in other countries. However, partnership with the Eurasian Medical Education Program would be the first example of an action-oriented program abroad. This turned out to be a highly advantageous relationship that brought considerable benefits to both parties. The ACP became an asset in recruiting expert physicians to travel to Russia and a respected source of curricular materials. Most of all, the ACP was held in high professional regard by our Russian colleagues.

The pattern adopted early was the recruitment of American and some western European physicians who would travel to Russia pro bono (expenses but no fees). Criteria for their selection included recognized professional knowledge and accomplishment in particular clinical areas, recognition as excellent teachers, and previous experience in foreign medical cultures. A few spoke Russian. Lectures would be delivered generally in English with sequential translation. Visual materials and written materials would be made available in the Russian language.

3

The Gestation Period: 1995 to 1997

Beyond the initial concept, development of the program required roughly two more years. That time was devoted to establishing partnership arrangements in Russian medical centers, settling on the format of professional interactions, establishing administrative arrangements and reaching understandings and terms of agreements with Russian medical centers and, most important, arranging for financial support.

Several events occurred during this period that turned out to be highly beneficial to the eventual program. One of these was a series of early trips to centers in the Russian Far East in cooperation with the University of Alaska. Shortly following the breakup up of the Soviet Union, the University of Alaska, with the encouragement of the late Senator Ted Stevens, established the American-Russian Center to encourage commerce across the Bering Straits and to bring American business practices to Russia. In behalf of this project, the University of Alaska established four centers in the Russian Far East—Republic of Sakha (Yakutia), Magadan, Khabarovsk, and Yuzhno-Sakhalinsk. In 1994, the physician community in Sakha (Yakutia) prevailed upon the University of Alaska to provide some advisors to acquaint the Russian community with successful models of medical organization and financing. The Russian Federation had just introduced a new constitution in 1993 and a new health insurance law, which aimed at partially financing medicine from payroll taxes. One result of the latter was to distribute a large portion of financial resources for health to the regions. But anticipation of this change was the cause of much concern among practicing physicians.

Remuneration for physician services and support of medicine generally appeared increasingly precarious. As a result, the founders of the Eurasian Medical Education Program were recruited to travel in March 1995 to Yakutsk, the capital of Sakha (Yakutia), to spend ten days in lectures and discussions of successful patterns of medical organization and financing in other parts of the world.

The Republic of Sakha(Yakutia) is six times the size of France, or about the land mass of western Europe. It stretches from the northern end of Lake Baikal to the Arctic Ocean but contains only one million inhabitants, a mixture of ethnic Russians and national minorities. The ethnic Russians are an interesting combination of historical circumstances—grandchildren of earlier explorers and fur traders, children of prisoners exiled to the Far East and, most recently, Russians lured to that part of the world by financial emoluments.

Yakutia is a major source of gem diamonds and gold. The Yakut government, having negotiated with Moscow its share of the revenue stream from diamond mining operations, had embarked on a series of ambitious social projects including housing and medical care. The per capita income of the residents was nearly twice that of the nation as a whole. Because of the far northern location of the capital, Yakutsk, the permafrost is two hundred meters deep. As one of the consequences, the traditional houses, constructed of massive, squared tamarack logs, have been sinking into the permafrost for years. First-floor windowsills are typically at ground level. Modern construction relies on elevating the first floor many feet above the ground to prevent the heat of the building from warming the permafrost surface below.

Because the only hotel was under reconstruction, we were installed in the Diagnostic Center—an ultramodern setting built only a few years earlier by an Austrian firm. Its design conformed to the far north construction practice of isolation from the ground.

In Sakha-Yakutia we encountered several instances of a never-ending series of humorous and paradoxical discoveries in Russia. First, we noticed that a small building adjacent to the Yakutsk airport was still named the Lend-Lease Building -- a reference to the period when the United States supplied aircraft to Russia during World War II, typically flying them to Yakutia from Nome Alaska.

As a side issue, I had been asked by the National Institutes of Health to combine this educational trip with a task associated with an unusual neurological disease, Vilius encephalomyelitis. This neurological disease was endemic in the vicinity of the Viliui River, near the capital city. It was believed to be of infectious origin, but the causative agent was unclear. The National Institute of Neurological Disorders and Stroke, a part of the U.S. National Institutes of Health (NIH), had undertaken a collaborative research project to learn more about this disease. I was asked by NIH to return from Yakutia with an insulated box containing brain tissue samples packed in dry ice for further study at NIH. That mission proceeded without incident until we were stopped at the departure gate of the airport in Moscow. The specimen then had to be transported back across the country to be exited out of the Russian Far East to Alaska.

Finally, the weather was another source of wonderful cultural disconnects. The day of our departure from Yakutsk to Moscow, March 18, was recognized as the official end of winter. The temperature had risen to -36ºF. However, this low temperature did not limit human activity. The streets were filled with pedestrians. The accompanying photograph shows two elegantly dressed Russian women standing in an open air market, eating one Russians' favorite foods—ice cream.

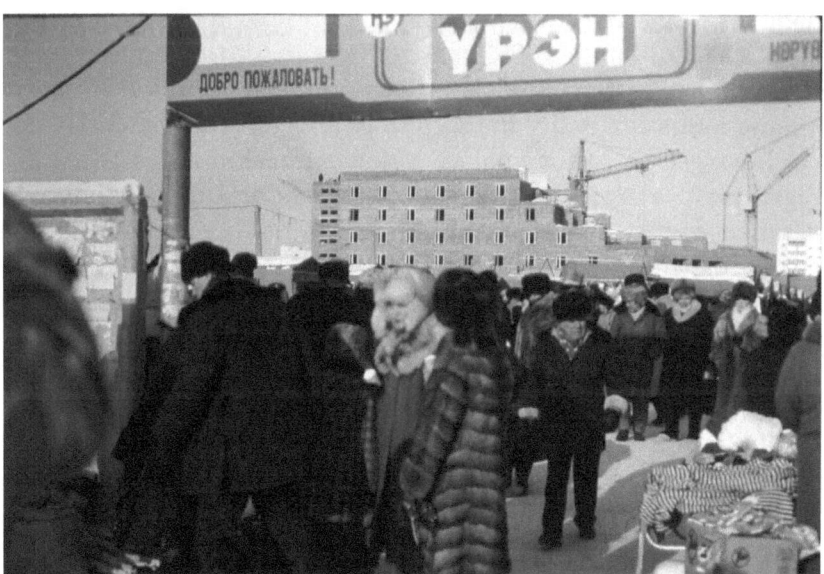

Women in fur coats in the open air market eating ice cream at -36°F.

We spent ten days in intensive seminar-like discussions with a great deal of back and forth interchange addressing the following issues:

- Provision of affordable care to all of the people
- Improvement of the quality of health care
- Management of costs, especially administrative costs
- Alternatives for a mixture of state and private health care delivery systems
- Alternative patterns of organization and financing of medical care
- Contrast between state-determined standards of care in Russia and the role of the professions in the United States

Our experience in Sakha-Yakutia was apparently well received because the two of us were asked to return a few weeks later for a repeat performance in Yuzhno-Sakhalinsk, the capital of Sakhalin Oblast. Sakhalin is a six-hundred-mile-long island lying east of the mainland of Russia. The area is physically beautiful with two north-south mountain ranges and a great many freshwater lakes, but it was economically depressed. It claims a very interesting history, reflecting wars and treaties in the Far East. Anton Chekhov made his way across Russia to Sakhalin in 1890 in his study of prisons. As a result of the 1905 Treaty of Portsmouth, which settled the Russo-Japanese War, the island was politically divided in half; it became a Russian entity in its entirety after World War II. The former Japanese governor's palace is now a museum.

We held a series of intensive seminars and discussions with members of the physician community over a three-day period. As in Yakutia, topics concentrated on organization of medical care, patterns of financing, and the prominent roles of the profession and professional societies in education, standards setting, and certification.

The majority of questions turned around financing. By now, the new health insurance law was in place, although the Sakhalin Oblast government had elected to adopt the new law gradually. During the three to four months prior to our arrival, physicians had not received any salary. Pensions would deliver only $45 to $50 per month. One spokesman observed that as many as 30% of the physicians would find themselves with no job. In spite of the depressed economy, there was anticipation of improvement with the prospect of extensive oil and gas reserves at the north end of the island.

The early decision to concentrate the Eurasian Medical Education Program in regions of Russia rather than in the major population centers turned out to be of enormous importance for the effectiveness and success of the program. The regions selected were marked by substantial technical strengths. There was a strong desire to embrace professional exchanges. By avoiding Moscow, we bypassed the pronounced political overlay that inevitably marked transactions in that city. A further benefit of this strategy came from the revised pattern of health care financing in Russia. The new health insurance law of 1993 was based on a withholding tax of 3.6%. The law directed that the majority of the tax, 3.4%, would not flow back to Moscow but would reside in "obligatory health insurance funds" in each region to support salaries and services. The remaining 0.2% would be returned to Moscow, but not to the Russian Federation Ministry of Health. This arrangement had an immediate effect of redistributing a substantial portion of funding centrifugally, increasing to some extent the power of the regions.

In 1996, I met with the Russian Federation Ministry of Health in Moscow and explained the sense of the then-proposed Eurasian Medical Education Program. The Ministry's response was an offer to set up a task force to assist the program. We did not press the Ministry to follow up on its offer. In fact, we independently selected an initial five geographic regions on the basis of the professional reputation of the academic medical center in each region and an expression by the medical and political leadership there of a desire for the program.

We established the individual cooperative agreements and memoranda of understanding with the regional authorities by personally approaching the medical and political leaders in each case. These approaches always returned a positive and enthusiastic invitation for cooperation, reflecting a strong desire for reestablishment of professional interaction following years of isolation. The partnership with the American College of Physicians carried high respect.

Early in this period, I joined a five-person Health Trade Mission to Russia sponsored by the U.S. Department of Commerce. The overall goal of this mission was to explore business opportunities in the pharmaceutical and medical device sectors in two regions, Nizhny Novgorod and Kazan, and to test the receptivity among the political and medical leadership for a cooperative program in postgraduate medical education. Thus, over a nine-day period, the delegation held discussions in Moscow, Nizhny Novgorod, and Kazan. One of our numbers, Michael Herzen, then a resident of California, was the great-grandson of Alexander Herzen, a famous nineteenth century Russian writer and thinker.

In the two regional centers, the delegation visited hospitals, polyclinics, and manufacturing firms. We met at length with regional governors and academic medical leaders. In each case, I would present the concept of a two-way, cooperative program, including physician exchanges for the purpose of sharing knowledge and experience. What was apparent in these visits was a strong desire to embrace professional contacts and learn about contemporary understanding of the management of disease. Ultimately, one of these regions, Tatarstan, was incorporated into the program of the Eurasian Medical Education Program.

The initial five regional academic medical centers selected for the program were Tula; Kazan; Ekaterinburg; and two regions in the Russian Far East, Khabarovsk and Birobidzhan.

Tula, 125 miles south of Moscow, was the home of Leo Tolstoy and was known as the samovar capital of Russia and the location of a small armament facility. The medical academic affiliation was with the Moscow Medical Academy.

Ekaterinburg, the capital of Sverdlovsk Oblast in the Ural Mountains, a large industrial center, is the birthplace of Boris Yeltsin and the site of the assassination of the last czar. The Ural State Medical University was considered outstanding with a particular contribution to the management of infectious diseases, including tuberculosis.

Kazan, the capital of the Republic of Tatarstan, is located on the Volga River, roughly five hundred miles east of Moscow. The city is physically beautiful with much attractive, old architecture reflecting its history as a prosperous Volga port. Kazan is one of then twenty-one semiautonomous republics within the Russian Federation enjoying an extra degree of political autonomy in governance. Notably, half of the population of Tatarstan is Muslim (Tatars). The remarkable aspect was the striking harmony between the Muslim and Orthodox sects. Much of this was said to be due to a longstanding political leader, President Mintimer Shaimiev. Symptomatic of this remarkable harmony, a mosque was constructed within the walls of the kremlin (citadel) of the city. Kazan claimed two academic medical teaching facilities—the Kazan State Medical Academy, devoted to postgraduate training, and the Kazan State Medical University. The cardiovascular physicians had already built and equipped a very impressive, new regional cardiovascular center, partly completed with backing from the U.S. Export-Import Bank.

Khabarovsk, on the Amur River in the Russian Far East, also boasted a well-respected medical and academic leadership. The Khabarovsk Krai is looked to as a leading center of the Far East. Its capital lies approximately 250 miles north of Vladivostok. The faculty of the Far Eastern Medical University was of high standing.

Birobidzhan is the capital of the Jewish Autonomous Region which was the product of a Stalin policy of concentrating Jews in that area . Street signs are in both Cyrillic and Hebrew. Currently, only about 2% of the population is Jewish. Birobidzhan was chosen to be one of the first five regions because of its high level of tuberculosis and the fact that it includes a prison. The medical community looks to Khabarovsk about a three-hour east, for its academic connection.

Our initial reception in nearly every case was one of warm welcome. At the same time, our hosts indicated a concern that the first visit would not be our last. Continuity of this endeavor over a prolonged period of time, not unexpectedly, turned out to be of great importance. Well-meaning individual physicians, church groups, and hospitals had already built a reputation of single visits. The pattern we adopted of returning became an important element in the success of the program.

The program quickly settled into a pattern of bringing one to three physician experts to each center for a period of one to two weeks. The sessions were in part didactic and, in many cases, seminars and discussion in form. Active participation and questioning by members of the physician audience in an academic setting was not traditional in Russia. We broke that pattern by encouraging active challenging and questioning. We always scheduled at least one session of clinical teaching rounds including at patients' bedside.

The choices of clinical subjects were made in consultation with our hosts. In general, however, we tended to concentrate on four clinical areas: cardiovascular disease, diabetes, tuberculosis, and HIV/AIDS. These were among the major contributors to premature or excess mortality in Russia and were amenable to medical intervention. From time to time, there were some important further additions. The rector of the medical university in Khabarovsk, on his own initiative, had established a department and a training program for family medicine. At his request, the Eurasian Medical Education Program brought one of the United States' best experts on family medicine to collaborate on that subject.

The administrative arrangements adopted were, by design, very simple. A staff of five in Washington included three physicians plus financial and administrative persons. An important element was the contribution of one or two Russian-speaking interns. The key, however, was the pattern of appointing and reimbursing, in most of the Russian regions, a person to serve as program coordinator. In general, these were young or middle-aged physicians, recommended by the medical center leadership, who had the respect of the faculty in each case. They performed two important functions: they could deal effectively with the academic hierarchy, and they were responsible for simple administrative tasks, such as scheduling and accommodations.

Financial Support

Simultaneous with developing the program and establishing the understandings and cooperative arrangements with the Russian centers, a strategy for financial support was established. From the beginning, as a principle, the founders were determined to see the program maintained by a balance of private and governmental support. This strategy achieved a level of funding approaching $1 million per year. An important element was an early grant of nearly $2 million from the Bill and Melinda Gates Foundation. This was followed by additional support from other foundations and from individuals who were interested in U.S.-Russian relations and saw Russian demographic trends and social instability as security issues.

U.S. federal government support became a challenge of a different sort. We recognized a parallel between the goals and strategies of the Eurasian Medical Education Program and those of a similar program concerned with the rule of law. Somewhat earlier, the leadership of the American Bar Association put in place a program initially known as the Central and East European Law Initiative (CEELI). That program, designed to encourage an effective and independent judiciary, brought pro bono professors of law and judges to various centers in Russia. The funding was almost entirely from the U.S. Agency for International Development. The parallel with our own program in medical education seemed obvious.

The founders of the Eurasian Medical Education Program proposed an early meeting with one of the senior spokesmen for USAID to outline the goals of the program, the strategy proposed, the partnership with the American College of Physicians, and the opportunity to enjoy the active participation of some America's most highly recognized medical talent. The initial response to that inquiry was lack of interest. Subsequently, it was apparent that USAID was not enamored by the prospect of voluntary contributions, entertained something of an aversion to clinical medicine, and was not interested in initiatives that originated outside the agency.

That response left two alternatives—retreat or go to Congress. We chose the latter. As a result, the State, Foreign Operations, and Related Programs Subcommittee of the U.S. Senate Appropriations Committee became a strong and consistent supporter of the program for the next fifteen years, realizing the value of medical diplomacy it represented and its potential for engagement with Russia. The result was an immediate reversal of USAID's position and a year-by-year support by the agency over the next fifteen years.

The relationship with USAID might be described as one of constructive tension. The agency influenced the choice of regions to be visited. The Eurasian Medical Education Program participated actively in periodic reviews of USAID's and other donors' reviews of investments and strategies in Russia. The program was subjected to never-ending changes in political thinking on emphasis and focus in Russia. A frequent disagreement occurred over emphasis on clinical subjects and diseases. The overwhelming political focus dictated by USAID was on HIV/AIDS. This overshadowed any logical ranking of importance. Hence, maintaining a balance between concentration on AIDS or on heart attacks and stroke (the latter overwhelmingly the principal impacts on Russian health and amenable to prevention and treatment) was a constant struggle.

4

The Program

An early desire of the architects of the Eurasian Medical Education Program was to concentrate its proposed activity in the regions of Russia. The rationale was straightforward. It appeared advantageous to avoid an inevitable overlay of political interests in Moscow and St. Petersburg. Perhaps most important, we guessed (correctly) that we would find substantial medical and scientific strengths in selected medical academic centers. Additionally, we hoped for a positive reception and cooperation from the corresponding regional political leadership. We were rewarded unequivocally in both cases.

While we recognized that a regional focus was a main orientation of the program, initial overtures were made in Moscow to the Russian Federation Ministry of Health and the Moscow State Medical Academy. Thus, in 1998, meetings were held with key members of the Ministry of Health on four occasions between May and September. This initial series of meetings lasted ten days with members from the Ministry of Health and other professional colleagues and academic medical leaders from two of the Russian centers chosen as initial sites for the programs. The general purpose of these meetings was to consider with the Ministry the design of the program, the choice of regions and the regional academic medical centers, and the necessary administrative arrangements.

The core of the program, as designed, was a visit to each regional academic medical center in groups of one to three physicians specializing in internal medicine for periods of one to two weeks. The visiting expert physicians would engage in lectures, discussions, and clinical teaching rounds with patients. Visiting physicians would be chosen on the basis of their recognized contribution to medicine, reputation as excellent teachers, and experience in foreign medical cultures. Some spoke Russian. The American College of Physicians would assist in the recruiting of candidates. Visiting physicians would be reimbursed for expenses but not receive any fees.

The Ministry urged that the program emphasize the importance of therapeutic interventions for which there was an empirical basis. This emphasis on "evidence-based medicine" clearly reflected concern over the rapid adoption of medical procedures in Russia over the past seventy years for which there was no basis in fact. We saw many examples over the course of the program.

These discussions emphasized the importance of primary versus specialist medical care. The Russian medical system, as in the United States, suffered from an emphasis on specialists and professional deference to specialists, often hospital-based. The reliance on specialists, combined with rather rigid compartmentalization of disease interests, made integration of care difficult. Primary care physicians were expected to treat uncomplicated hypertension. Diabetes, however, would fall to the realm of endocrinologists. Physicians treating AIDS were apart from those managing tuberculosis, even though the diseases commonly occurred together.

The Ministry placed a great deal of importance on leverage that could accrue from the program. That is, the Ministry hoped that the didactic material we provided could be made available to medical postgraduate education settings in addition to those where we had established programs.

Finally, we discussed the importance of evaluation of our program measured both as comprehension and as appropriate influence on physician practice patterns.

These initial presentations and discussions were enthusiastically received. The spokesmen for the Ministry proposed appointing a task force to monitor and assist the program. We were asked to sign a formal memorandum of agreement. Professor Igor Denisov, Vice Rector for Academic Studies, Moscow Medical Academy, requested assistance from the program and the American College of Physicians in developing contemporary standards of care broadly for the Russian Federation.

In sum, the enthusiastic reception the program was given at the outset was outstanding and very encouraging. The point was underscored by a request to consider extending the initial program to many other parts of the Russian Federation.

Initial Trips Made to Ekaterinburg and Khabarovsk

Ekaterinburg, the capital of Sverdlovsk Oblast in the Ural Mountains, is an industrial city of 1.4 million people. Its early industries harnessed water power for steel making and mining of semiprecious stones from the Ural Mountains.

The Eurasian Medical Education Program was able to assume an earlier physician exchange arrangement between Ekaterinburg and the University of Rochester. The initial program coordinator was Dr. Alexei Sirotkin. Dr. Sirotkin would eventually move to the United States.

The initial meeting included Dr. Anatoli P. Yastrebov, rector of the Ural State Medical Academy, and Dr. Maria Syrochkina, assistant for international affairs (who would later serve as program coordinator for the region). Dr. Yastrebov exhibited strong support for the American College of Physicians initiative, with a particular interest in family medicine, acquisition of educational materials in both electronic and printed forms rendered into the Russian language, and provision for bringing physicians from Ekaterinburg to medical centers in the United States.

The discussions, which included several physicians from the academic medical institutions and hospitals, indicated strong support for the Eurasian Medical Education Program, its proposed format, and specific choices of disease entities to consider. A key individual was Dr. Yuri Chugaev, professor and chairman of the Tuberculosis Department. Tuberculosis and drug-resistant tuberculosis were prevalent in the Sverdlovsk Oblast. The infectious disease department was particularly strong.

This visit coincided with the Russian celebration of Victory Day on May 9. Russia recognizes this date as the point when the Russian forces marched into Berlin, ending World War II. That date trumps all other holidays in Russia. Our Russian program coordinator, while heroically searching for a restaurant for dinner, declared, "Well, we'll have to put up with long-legged women." The ultimate choice for dinner turned out to be a crowded casino. We were forced to check our cameras at the door lest we capture compromising scenes.

The program expanded from Ekaterinburg to the city of Khabarovsk in the Russian Far East. Khabarovsk, with its population of 590,000, was established as a military outpost in the 1880s and gained further notoriety in the book and film entitled *Dersu Uzala*. The city is located approximately 250 miles north of Vladivostok with commanding views of the Amur River.

The initial American delegation of three persons spent an intense two days of discussions with the medical and political leadership of Khabarovsk. Key among these were Dr. Boris Kogut, director of the Far Eastern State Medical University; Dr. Tatyana Polyakova, medical director, Public Health Department; and Irina Strelkova, deputy governor of the Khabarovsk Krai. Mrs. Strelkova remained a strong supporter of the program throughout the next fifteen years. Also joining the meetings were Dr. Nikolay Kapitolinko, director of the Khabarovsk Krai Medical Insurance Fund, and Dr. Vladimir Bishovsky, professor and chairman of the Department of Family Medicine.

A key to the arrangements in the city was Anatoli Fomine. Mr. Fomine had formerly been assistant to the governor of the Khabarovsk Krai and more recently a Humphrey Fellow at the University of Texas. Anatoli Fomine was appointed as program coordinator for Khabarovsk and for activities in other parts of the Russian Far East. Dr. Boris Kogut, rector of the medical university in Khabarovsk, had initiated a program of service and teaching in the field of family medicine. Over the subsequent years, the Eurasian Medical Education Program would engage the family medicine program in a number of cooperative ways.

Dr. Kogut, together with several of the key medical leadership, met with us, first to warmly welcome and endorse the proposed cooperative program and also to pose some searching questions:

- Would the program deal with clinical medical subjects or with administrative issues?
- Would it concentrate on clinical medical practice or on medical technologies?

- Would it have an interest in family medicine and primary care?
- What was the state and solidity of funding?
- How long would the project be expected to last?

We were apprised of a series of former or existing relationships with other American medical institutions, including the University of Oregon, the University of Kentucky, and Washington and Virginia Mason Hospital in Seattle. The sense of many of these inquiries was to determine how permanent a commitment we were proposing. It became evident that the element of continuity over a period of time (measured in years) was an extremely important criterion for acceptance.

The following month, a second meeting with the Ministry of Health brought agreement on the choice of clinical subjects, emphasis on evidence basis for medical practice, importance of evaluation of results, and a strong endorsement of the program. From that meeting in Moscow, we established the center in Kazan.

There are two academic medical institutions in Kazan—the Kazan State Medical University and the Kazan State Medical Academy. Over two days, we met with the leadership of both institutions together with key clinical faculty, discussing diabetes, cardiovascular disease, and tuberculosis. The purpose of these meetings once again was to review the burden of disease in the region, problem areas, available resources and programs for control, and the character of current professional educational efforts. The postgraduate education provided to general internists and chest physicians was found to be well developed in Kazan. Physicians are subject to periodic continuing medical education through short courses and two-month full-time courses.

Dr. Lilia Ziganshina agreed to serve as program coordinator. This remarkable individual was the youngest full professor ever appointed to the medical academy. Specializing in clinical pharmacology, she served the Eurasian Medical Education Program with outstanding distinction for the next fifteen years. The initial meeting in Kazan emerged with a tentative schedule of follow-on visits.

A month later, we held a third series of meetings in Moscow with the Russian Federation Ministry of Health. Dr. Igor Denisov, Moscow Medical Academy, used the meeting to make a series of points:

- The Russians would like to see educational materials for three categories of individuals:
  — Materials for polyclinic practitioners
  — Guidelines for nursing personnel
  — Materials for patients
- There was a plea for concentration on basic medical educational materials.
- There was an interest in electronic forms of educational materials (e.g., CDs, audiotapes).
- The program should be treated as a cooperative affair with Russians serving as collaborators in the choice and review of materials.
- The program should concentrate on reducing cerebrovascular accidents (stroke).

After the Moscow meeting we traveled to Tula to explore with the leadership there the adoption of that region as a fourth site for the program. The City of Tula is 107 miles south of Moscow. It looks to the Moscow Medical Academy for its tie to the academic medical world.

A key individual in the meeting was Dr. Victor Aleksandrovich Melnikov, deputy director, Tula Oblast Department of Health. We met with twenty physicians, administrators, and computer specialists from the Tula Oblast. The discussions focused on cardiovascular disease and, in particular, on hypertension. An estimated 27% of the population is hypertensive (a prevalence common in other parts of the world); however, only 8% of hypertensives are recognized. The representatives from Tula endorsed the proposed program of the American College of Physicians. Dr. Melnikov offered himself as program coordinator.

In October 1998, we held a fourth set of meetings in Moscow with the Russian Federation Ministry of Health. As a request from the Ministry, we had prepared a series of draft curricula for review. The Moscow Medical Academy senior faculty strongly supported the draft documents. This was followed by a discussion that underscored the importance of collaboration in the development of curricula, concentration on material for generalist physicians, and encouragement of collaboration between regional medical universities and postgraduate medical academies. This again urged a cooperative spirit between the Eurasian Medical Education Program and Russian counterparts.

Thus, the Eurasian Medical Education Program was given a warm and enthusiastic reception by the Russian Federation Ministry of Health at the outset. The meetings established a sense of professional collaboration and acknowledged the potential for contribution in both directions and agreement on areas of particular emphasis. Finally, they encouraged continual communication with the program.

In practice, while maintaining nominal ties to the Federation Ministry of Health, the Eurasian Medical Education Program focused increasingly on its relations with regional political and medical leadership. This was the result of several factors. One was the frequent change of leadership within the Federal Ministry. Over the seventeen years of the active period of the Eurasian Medical Education Program, there was a succession of federal ministers of health. Other factors made the regional strategy of the program increasingly attractive. The regional leaders with whom we developed individual memoranda of agreement all became strongly enthusiastic about the development of cooperative professional arrangements. As a result, their generosity was remarkable.

Thus began a series of professional missions to regional medical centers over the next fifteen years. The original five regions (Tula, Kazan, Ekaterinburg, Khabarovsk, and Birobidzhan) were eventually expanded to thirteen geographic regions reaching from the Leningrad Oblast to Yuzhno-Sakhalinsk (Sahkalin Island) - spanning most of the eleven time zones of Russia. Generally, at the request of our Russian hoss, we added a few additional clinical subjects to the original three. These included family medicine, inflammatory bowel disease. osteoporosis and women's health. The core program remained fairly constant. Visiting expert internists would travel to each center in groups of one to three to spend typically a week in intensive interaction with Russian colleagues to review and discuss contemporary understanding of clinical management of disease and standards of care. Russian audiences ranged from 20 to 250. Printed materials and visual materials (PowerPoint slides) were provided in Russian. Sequential translation was available for lectures and discussions. When possible, the sessions were scheduled to coincide with the Russians' continuing medical education courses. This permitted American exposure to Russian experience and standards of care.

With the assistance of the American College of Physicians, the program recruited fifty of some of the most highly recognized American experts to travel to Russia multiple times. Nearly all of them held academic titles. Examples were Dr. Gerald Bernstein, professor of medicine and president of the American Diabetes Association, Dr Sara Walker, professor of medicine, University of Missouri, and president of the American College of Physicians; Dr. Michael Iseman, The Gerald and Madeline Beno Chair in Mycobacterial Disease, National Jewish Medical and Research Center, Denver, Colorado; and Dr. Donna Sweet, professor of Medicine, University of Kansas, Wichita, Kansas. The recognized professional accomplishments of these experts were of no little importance in the Russians' respect for the program.

In November and December 1998, the program spent a week in Tula concerned with cardiovascular disease and hypertension, another week in Ekaterinburg focused on tuberculosis, and a third trip to Kazan. This was a period of severe economic downturn in Russia. The Russian ruble was devalued from 1 RUB/USD to 22 RUB/USD. An overnight train trip between Kazan and Moscow found factory workers on the station platforms selling the very products they had been engaged in manufacturing as a source of money. This was also the period during which Russians experienced severe letdown and some hostility following their initial enthusiasm for a market economy in the first years of the 1990s. None of that shift in outlook influenced the course of the Eurasian Medical Education Program.

In February 1999, the program visited Ekaterinburg. The subject was the management of complications of diabetes. Visits to three hospitals revealed state-of-the art equipment and knowledgeable endocrinologists. As would be revealed in later visits, management of diabetes is referred to endocrinologists rather than primary care physicians.

In September 1999, I met at some length with Dr. Evgeny Chazov, director general, Cardiology Research Center, in Moscow. Dr. Chazov had been the Russian overseer of what began in 1972 as the Joint U.S.-Soviet Cardiopulmonary Research Program. I had helped to foster this program with the National Heart, Lung, and Blood Institute of NIH during the period of détente. Dr. Chazov had served as federal minister of health for about three years and, in that position, had become something of a stern critic of the Russian health care system. On the issue of education of physicians, Dr. Chazov's conviction was that Russian physicians at the top of the hierarchy were well trained and as capable as any in cardiovascular disease. He felt, however, that midlevel physicians were the ones in need of additional exposure to educational material and seminars.

Just after midnight, I flew from Moscow to Novosibirsk and to two centers in the Russian Far East—Khabarovsk and Yuzhno-Sakhalinsk. This began a several-years-long period of cooperation with Rotary International. At that point, there were seventy Rotary clubs in Russia, most of which were located in Siberia and the Russian Far East. Because of Steven Yoshida, an energetic Rotarian in Alaska and a former district governor, Rotary clubs in the eastern part of Russia had been engaged to develop health fairs in those communities. Thus, less than a decade after the end of the Cold War, the Eurasian Medical Education Program found itself in the company of Rotarians who resembled in every way their counterparts in middle America. As a result, exploratory visits to academic medical centers and the regional political leadership were combined with a series of functions associated with Rotary. In the course of this trip, I was the beneficiary of extraordinary generosity and witness to wonderful ironies that characterize contemporary Russia.

In Novosibirsk, I enjoyed the personal hospitality of Alexander Mouzychenko and his family. Mr. Mouzychenko had an advanced degree in oceanography. With the collapse of the Soviet Union, he turned away from science to business by providing financial information to clients and serving as a representative for the legal research organization, LexisNexis, for Siberia and the Russian Far East.

A further visit in Novosibirsk was to the Vector Laboratory (State Research Center of Virology and Biotechnology (VECTOR), the premier closed city research and production facility for biological warfare agents. Following the end of the Soviet Union, the Vector Laboratory had been actively seeking new, nonmilitary outlets for its scientific prowess and professional resources. By the time of our visit, 40% of the scientific personnel had departed. Strengths in the laboratory were virology, vaccine development, and physical facilities for both animal and human trials. The purpose of this visit was to explore the possibility of a satellite-based videoconferencing facility for distance learning for the Novosibirsk Medical Academy and to examine the possibility of using the Vector Laboratory facilities for tuberculosis testing in Novosibirsk.

A few days with Rotarians in Khabarovsk were equally fascinating. Because of a change in travel plans, I arrived in Khabarovsk with no prearranged lodging. I was immediately taken into an apartment by a Rotarian, Victor Smolyak, his wife, and mother.Mr. Smolyak had been a renowned political economist and academician (chairman, Department of Social and Economic Problems of Foreign Countries, Institute of Economic Research). He had been a member of the Soviet Academy of Sciences and had intermediated a large number of international exchanges. More recently he had been a well-known political commentator on nationwide Russian television until his criticism of the federal government caused his dismissal. Yet, he was contributing occasional pieces to *Izvestia*. His wife taught philosophy at a local institution. Their combined pensions amounted to $40 a month.

In Yuzhno-Sakhalinsk, we were housed in a very different but unusual setting. We were billeted with the family employed by the Sakhalin Energy Company in a gated community that appeared straight out of suburban America. Meetings with the health leadership eventually led to the adoption of Yuzhno-Sakhalinsk as an additional region for the program.

This trip was designed as a step toward a hoped-for Rotary Foundation grant for health in the Russian Far East and Siberia. As program director, I was asked to speak at a large Rotary function in Seattle a few months hence. I wrote the speech for the president of Rotary International to deliver at that meeting. It became apparent that Rotary International holds limited influence over priorities of individual Rotary clubs. We did not succeed in receiving a grant.

The Eurasian Medical Education Program proceeded over the next twelve years to bring expert physicians trained in internal medicine to share experience and knowledge with colleagues in the Russian regional centers. Over this period as well, eight additional regions were added to the original five, mostly at the invitation of the medical leadership in those regions. The first was Centers that followed included Sakha-Yakutia, Irkutsk, Blagoveshchensk, Khanty-Mansiysk, Novosibirsk, Vladivostok, and the Leningrad Oblast (the territory surrounding the city of St. Petersburg).

Noncommunicable Disease

As noted at the beginning, the program, in consultation with our Russian partners, endeavored to concentrate on clinical areas (diseases) recognized as the most prominent contributors to excess or premature mortality where medical intervention could make a difference. Following this guide, cardiovascular disease was clearly the most important candidate. Although the political spotlight was more often on the global burden of mortality associated with malaria, tuberculosis, and HIV/AIDS, cardiovascular disease caused more than three times the number of deaths than those other diseases combined. Cigarette smoking, elevated blood pressure, and blood lipids are all recognized as the most important risk factors leading to the development of heart attacks and stroke.[1]

One of the most important issues for the Russian economy and health in the early 1990s was demographic decline. Russia's population was declining at a rate of four hundred thousand to six hundred thousand persons per year net of any in-migration. The background was straightforward. The Russian Federation was experiencing more deaths than births. Fertility declined, and there was an excess in mortality—especially mortality of males in their most productive years. During the early part of the 1990s, male longevity from birth dropped to as low as fifty-seven years. As a result, Russia's population, 149 million in 1992, dropped to 143 million in 2003. Russia's total life expectancy lagged that in Japan by sixteen years and that of the European Union by fourteen years. There was also a fourteen-year difference between male and female longevity.

Noncommunicable diseases and injuries were the leading causes of death and sickness in Russia. Cardiovascular disease was the principal contributor to this statistic.[2] Mortality rates from noncommunicable disease were three times those in the European Union. Russia's cardiovascular disease death rate, 994 per one hundred thousand population in 2002, was one of the world's highest. Table 2 illustrates the specific cardiovascular mortality in the working age population in seven countries.

Table 2. Cardiovascular disease death rates per 100,000 among persons ages 33–64

	Country						
	South Africa	Brazil	China	India	Russia	United States	Portugal
Males	96.9	71.0	37.9	81.0	258.6	55.9	57.7
Females	68.2	48.9	23.8	55.9	63.7	27.9	17.9

Source: Mark G. Field, "The Physician in the Commonwealth of Independent States: The Difficult Passage from Bureaucrat to Professional," in *The Changing Medical Profession: An International Perspective*, ed. Frederic W. Hafferty and John B. McKinley (New York: Oxford University Press, 1993).

Ironically, demographic decline and, behind it, excess cardiovascular mortality were recognized early by the political leadership of the country. President Putin, in repeated reports to the nation and the Duma, referred to the problem and labeled it a serious security risk. However, there appeared little or no effective follow-up by the Ministry of Health.

Cardiovascular disease was a centerpiece of the Eurasian Medical Education Program in nearly all of the regions served. It was a subject of particular concentration in three of the regions—Kazan, Ekaterinburg, and Khabarovsk. In part, this was a reflection of the clinical skills and interests in place in these regions. In conjunction with continuing medical education, these centers were sites for active, directed demonstration programs of intervention and careful review of results.

Risk factor reduction was the goal. A particular focus was hypertension. Recognition of elevated blood pressure and interventions to reduce blood pressure were key elements in a strategy to reduce cardiovascular disease and mortality. Dramatic successes had been reported in western Europe in reducing cardiovascular mortality through attention to the risk factors responsible—especially hypertension.[3] Hence, early in the history of the Eurasian Medical Education Program, programs were established to reduce blood pressure in three regions of the Russian Federation—Tatarstan, Sverdlovsk, and Khabarovsk. These involved recognition of elevated blood pressure among patients in polyclinic settings who presented themselves with any complaint. Charts of these patients were followed over a three-year period. Management included pharmacologic interventions, follow-up attention to blood pressure, attention to complications, and patient education. Patient compliance with medication was a notable obstacle. The experience of these efforts did prove the effectiveness of a program to reduce the force of risk factors among patients in an ambulatory setting.[4]

We followed cohorts of recognized diabetes patients. In this case, the Russian state provided a notable advantage. Registration of a patient with recognized diabetes obligated the patient's follow-up and assured state-provided medication. Registration meant that a program could capture close to 100% of all diabetics in a region. Attention was given to control of diabetes and to reduction of complications of diabetes (diabetic foot, ocular disease, ketoacidosis, and neurologic complications). An interesting finding for both hypertension and diabetes programs was a tendency of Russian physicians to underdose medications, in part because of a concern for adverse side effects.

We were particularly fortunate to have some excellent professional endocrine collaboration. One of these was Professor Alexei Sirotin, Khabarovsk State Medical University, recognized as distinguished scientist in Russia.

Tuberculosis

Tuberculosis, a disease caused by a bacterial pathogen associated with artistic genius in the Romantic era and often featured in opera and literature, is a major challenge in Russia. tuberculosis was the most common cause of death in Russia between 1890 and 1940. Humans are the only known host. Traditionally, the disease was associated with poverty and overcrowding and particularly afflicted the elderly. By marked contrast, active tuberculosis in Russia in the 1990s was most prominent among the young and middle-aged. The disease had been taken seriously in the first and third Soviet five-year plans between 1932 and 1941, which brought money and facilities to the challenge.

Table 3. Antituberculosis facilities in Moscow, 1929 and 1939

Institutions and facilities	1929	1939
Tuberculosis dispensaries	12	13
TB departments in unified dispensaries and polyclinics	2	28
TB offices in enterprises	0	5
TB hospital beds, Department of Public Health	915	1,903

Source: Michael C. David, *Problems of Tuberculosis* 18, no. 12 (1940): 98.

Russia also adopted as a standard the antituberculosis Bacillus Calmette Guerin (BCG) vaccine, which has been shown to have effectiveness when given to the newborn. The Russian standard recommends three or more doses up through the age of twenty-seven absent a showing of efficacy.

Tuberculosis in Russia is commonly a parallel diagnosis with HIV infection. Finally, tuberculosis in prisons remains a particularly serious problem. The incidence and prevalence among prisoners are much higher than in the civilian population. Prisoners

Table 4. Tuberculosis incidence, prevalence, and mortality rates in Russian Federation, 2007

Variable	General population	HIV-infected individuals
Incidence		
All forms of TB (thousands per year)	157	26
All forms of TB (per 100,000 population)	110	18
Prevalence		
All forms of TB (thousands per year)	164	13
All forms of TB (per 100,000 population)	115	9
Mortality		
All forms of TB (thousands per year)	25	5.1
All forms of TB (per 100,000 population)	18	3.5
Mortality from drug-resistant TB		
Among all new TB cases (%)	13	
Among previously treated TB cases (%)	49	

Source: World Health Organization *WHO Global Tuberculosis Control: Epidemiology, Strategy, Financing*, WHO Report WHO/HTM/TB/2009.411(Geneva: World Health Organization), 2009.

released from prison through amnesty or discharge are frequently not subject to effective follow-up. This puts persons who are infectious back on the street to become a serious source of new contacts.

The Eurasian Medical Education Program first encountered tuberculosis in 1999 in Kazan. Mortality from drug-resistant tuberculosis (MDRTB) was reported in 1999 to have increased from 2% to 16% in ten years. MDRTB is a disease due to a strain of *M. tuberculosis* resistant to at lleast two first-line drugs -- INH and Rifampin.

In Sverdlovsk, the prevalence of TB among prisoners in the Nizhny Tagil prison was particularly high. In 2000, the total number of incarcerated persons was forty thousand, of whom 20% were TB positive. Over the same period, the number of persons with active TB increased from 1,255 to 1,259. Of the 2,300 prisoners released in 2000, 1,000 had active TB at the time of releasel and more than 40% of those did not have follow-ups after leaving prison. We relied particularly heavily on two resources in the United States for the programs in tuberculosis—National Jewish Health (formerly National Jewish Medical and Research Center) in Denver, Colorado (Drs. Michael Iseman, Charles Daley, and Leonid Heifets); and the New Jersey Medical School (Dr. Lee B. Reichman) in Newark. Each of these individuals made multiple trips to TB centers in Russia and received groups of Russian TB physicians and microbiologists for longer periods in their own centers.

Tuberculosis in Russia presented some unusual challenges. Some of these were political; others derived from the professional culture of TB management long in place in Russia. The head of tuberculosis control for the country, Dr. Alexander Khomenko, unexpectedly died in 1999 during one of our visits. He had been considered a reasonable and technically sound leader. His place was immediately taken by Michael J. Perlman, director, Central TB Research Institute, Moscow. Dr. Perlman led a campaign against the use of the treatment developed and proposed with the World Health Organization (WHO) known as direct observation therapy short course (DOTS).

At a donors' meeting that brought together funders of TB programs in Russia and organizations actively engaged against tuberculosis, Dr. Perlman took the opportunity to offer highly critical views of WHO and western medical strategies for TB. He presented his evidence to show that Russian methods were ultimately more successful than western ones. A particular target had been the DOTS strategy, which required patients to receive TB medications in the presence of medical personnel in order to reduce the possibility of noncompliance.

Another issue was treatment of uncomplicated, simple (nonresistant) tuberculosis in an ambulatory setting. The Russian tradition had been to hospitalize TB patients for long periods of time (years). While this clearly appeared unnecessary and expensive to our U.S. colleagues, in Russia there emerged an economic basis for not backing away from that tradition. Physical inpatient facilities had been in place and staffed for a long period. There was a fear of unemployment for large numbers of staff if an alternative was chosen. Ultimately, we reached a compromise, which was short-term hospitalization followed by out-of-hospital follow-up.

An important issue was accurate and timely diagnosis and characterization of the causative TB organisms. Professor Michael Iseman and Leonid Heifets visited a number of TB facilities across the Russian Federation. Their recommendations were straightforward and rested on two important principles—effective case finding and effective management of active TB. Effective case finding depended on valid identification of the TB organism in suspected individuals and characterization of the organism through microbiological laboratory techniques to determine sensitivity to drugs. Failure and delay at this point was a major cause of drug-resistant disease. Identification and characterization had to be accomplished in a short time to be effective. The accepted pattern had been a typical delay of three to six months. The visiting TB experts strongly recommended the building of a centralized model microbiological TB laboratory for each region.

A second series of recommendations was for appropriate drug therapy. Traditional Russian management of tuberculosis was described as "individualized" treatment with wide variations and extensive use of surgery. At one point, one of our visiting experts was confronted by a surgeon who insisted that "you will never solve the tuberculosis problem without the use of surgery." Failure to hew to recognized effective drug therapy promised an increase in MDRTB and extremely drug-resistant TB (XDRTB), the latter refers to organisms to both first- and second-line TB drugs.

In the city of Irkutsk, the tuberculosis hospital was severely inadequate in all aspects. It was very old and unreconstructed. The physical facilities were outdated. The record rooms (which could be seen from the street) appeared to be piles of unfiled record folders stacked on top of each other. The hospital was overcrowded and did not meet the infection safety standards necessary for safe conditions for personnel. Cross-infection among patients appeared highly likely, and there was high possibility of "exchange" of drug-resistant strains in overcrowded wards.

The diagnostic laboratory resources were similarly inadequate. The turnaround time for reporting the laboratory's drug susceptibility was from three to six months—an enormous drawback in achieving an efficient program of management of the tuberculosis epidemic. The TB bacteriological services in the Irkutsk Oblast were handled by ten laboratories and some forty "seeding stations." Sputum specimens were processed in the stations, and the inoculated specimens were sent (with some delay) to the laboratories for identification and, in some case, characterization. For final evaluation, the inoculated cultures were sent to the oblast dispensary laboratory. The combined steps of this process added to the turnaround time, compromising the diagnostic process and increasing the probability of wrongful therapy and multidrug-resistant disease.

The Japanese government had underwritten the construction and furnishing of an ultramodern diagnostic center in Irkutsk. This center purveyed materials and devices for a wide variety of diagnostic procedures. A categorical list along with prices was posted in the main hall of the center. Among tests available were polymeric chain reaction (PCR) testing based on molecular biology for tuberculosis. The tuberculosis specialists in Irkutsk used the facility as a substitute for traditional bacteriological culture and sensitivity. PCR testing is properly used to amplify certain characteristics of bacteria being examined. It is very rapid; however, it cannot substitute for traditional methods of microbiological testing.

A particularly impressive program was the Novosibirsk Tuberculosis Research Institute (NTRI) in Novosibirsk, Siberia. The Eurasian Medical Education Program was invited by the leadership of the NTRI to sponsor a series of lectures on multidrug-resistant TB by an expert on the subject. Our candidate was Dr. Charles Daley, an internationally recognized expert on the management of multi-drug-resistant disease, from the National Jewish Medical and Research Institute.

The Novosibirsk Tuberculosis Research Institute is an impressive institution. With broad responsibilities for all three - service, research, and education, the institute was established in 1943 as a part of a movement by the Soviet government to relocate scientific and technical facilities east of the Ural Mountains. The territory for which it has responsibility is vast and includes all of the Siberian Federal Region (5.1 million square miles) and the Far Eastern Federal Region (6.2 million square miles).*

The combined "zone of responsibility" covers an area equivalent to 67% of the land mass of Russia. The total population served is 26.7 million people—nearly 20% of the Russian population. The director of NTRI, Professor Vladimir Krasnov, is highly regarded within his profession.

The burden of tuberculosis and drug-resistant tuberculosis in these two super regions was among the highest in the nation and exceeded those registered for the Russian Federation generally. Discussion and lectures over several days concerned:

- Contemporary methods of management of multidrug resistant tuberculosis
- Infection control
- Appropriate uses of surgery for tuberculosis

Table 5. The burden of disease and TB-associated mortality

Variable (per 100,000 population)	Siberian federal district	Far Eastern federal district	Russian Federation
TB mortality	28.5	24.4	15.6
TB incidence	121.5	139.5	77.2
TB prevalence	294.0	317.0	185.1

The third topic was fascinating. The Russian profession had accepted surgical interventions for TB disease as standard of care. Surgery for the disease in other parts of the industrialized world had declined to almost zero. In some of our interactions with the TB profession in other parts of Russia, we were admonished for not admitting the effectiveness of surgical intervention for tuberculosis.

*The political designation of Federal Region arose in the;1990s with the division of all of Russia intoseven super regions - a pattern developed to increase Kremlin control.

This was a matter of frequent heated discussion. The sessions in Novosibirsk were deliberate, nonconfrontational efforts to examine all of the recognized evidence-based indications for surgery with a discussion of complications, benefits, and records of results.

HIV/AIDS

The Eurasian Medical Education Program was first thrust into the challenge of HIV/AIDS in 2009. One of the program's funding sources, USAID, suddenly insisted on an almost exclusive emphasis on HIV/AIDS, overwhelming the program's initial principle of concentrating on the major clinical areas responsible for premature or excess mortality. This pressure remained for the remainder of the program's years in Russia.

AIDS first appeared in Russia in the mid-1980s; it mushroomed as an epidemic between 1996 and 1997.

Table 6. AIDS in Russia

	1995	2001
Registered new cases	<1,000	87,000
Total reported cases	<1,000	175,000

The available data on HIV/AIDS were subject to severe underreporting and inaccuracy, in part reflecting the lack of desire to acknowledge and manage the problem. The U.S. National Intelligence Council published a report in 2002 that predicted a prevalence of three to four million HIV-positive individuals in Russia by 2010. Russia and Ukraine stood out among all other countries surveyed.[5] AIDS was predicted by some to account for a decrease in Russia's GDP of over 4%.[6]

Risk groups and risk factors behind the epidemic were well recognized. The largest risk group was intravenous drug users, followed by sex workers and their partners, and men having sex with men. The prominence of intravenous drug use colored the views of both the Russian governmen and the medical profession concerning actions against the HIV problem. A huge element of stigma shaped official and professional. Drug use was considered a criminal and law enforcement issue. Indeed, a study in 2007 indicated that HIV/AIDS among prisoners was estimated to be between 0.8% and 4.76% and as high as 46% in St. Petersburg.[7] Coinfection and comorbidity of HIV and tuberculosis were remarkably common. One-half of all deaths among HIV individuals were due to tuberculosis.

While the Russian Federation government had chosen generally to ignore the AIDS epidemic, a series of international institutions—including the Joint United Nations Programme on HIV/AIDS (UNAIDS); the Global Fund for TB, Malaria and HIV/AIDS; and the World Bank—stepped up to the challenge. The U.S. government's view across several agencies (USAID, Department of State, the National Security Council) was mixed at first. By 2004, USAID's priority for Russia was fixed almost exclusively on HIV/AIDS. This had the perverse effect of shifting support away from the balance established by the Eurasian Medical Education Program.

The burden of HIV/AIDS in Irkutsk in 2009 was exceptionally high. Factors responsible for the high prevalence of HIV/AIDS were:

- Ignorance among many subjects concerning their HIV status
- Lack of understanding about risky behavior
- High level of intravenous drug use (50% of all drug users seeking treatment were found to be HIV-positive)
- Location of Irkutsk close to Russia's southern border and trade routes to Afghanistan
- Inclusion of eight prisons in the region

In March 2009 The Eurasian Medical Education Program brought to the Irkutsk Oblast Dr. Donna Sweet, University of Kansas Medical Center in Wichita. Dr. Sweet is recognized as one of America's principal AIDS experts. She had been chairman of the Board of Regents of the American College of Physicians and maintains a highly active practice at the University of Kansas. Once a week she traveled throughout the State of Kansas dealing with patients with AIDS. Dr. Sweet returned repeatedly to Russian centers across the Russian Federation to lecture and teach the profession about the prevention and management of AIDS.

Russian colleagues who joined Dr. Sweet's sessions in Irkutsk included AIDS specialists, infectious disease specialists, pediatricians, epidemiologists, representatives from the regional AIDS center, and representatives from the regional Ministry of Health. The continuing medical education sessions were divided among nine separate periods

- Basic science of HIV infection, incorporating the most current scientific information
- Recommended antiretroviral therapy (ART), including when to begin ART and risks associated with it.
- Pediatric HIV infection, prevention, differences between adults and children, and interpretation of laboratory results
- Hepatitis A and B and HIV infection
- HIV and hepatitis C
- HIV and tuberculosis—the characteristics and progression of TB diseasein the face of HIV, principles of treatment, drug-drug interactions
- HIV and cardiovascular disease
- Importance of traditional risk factors

For the next several years, the Eurasian Medical Education Program remained nearly exclusively focused on HIV/AIDS and tuberculosis, this despite the burden of cardiovascular morbidity and mortality and repeated requests by our Russian colleagues to treat those diseases. Most of the AIDS and TB work took place in academic medical centers in eastern Russia—particularly Siberia and the Russian Far East. The specific regions included Irkutsk, Novosibirsk, Yakutsk, Blagoveshchensk, Khabarovsk, and the Jewish Autonomous Region, as well as the Leningrad Oblast and Sverdlovsk. In addition, the program brought to centers in the United States a series of delegations of physicians and health leaders for more extensive experience in managing AIDS and tuberculosis. U.S. centers that served as hosts included Georgetown University, Johns Hopkins University, and the New Jersey Medical Center. Residence in these locations was typically two to four weeks and included clinical experience and laboratory diagnosis.

The program witnessed an interesting exercise in Khabarovsk designed to understand the origin of the HIV infectious agents, presumably reflecting human migratory patterns. Genotyping of HIV organisms collected from patients was performed, and the results were classified as to subtypes. Conclusions from this work indicated that HIV found in patients in Khabarovsk had migrated from western Russia. HIV found in Sakhalin had migrated from mainland Asia (Hong Kong and Vietnam).

There were a number of common features among the several AIDS programs. First and foremost was the effect of the stigma expressed against patients with AIDS and drug users This led to the separation of the clinical management of AIDS from the professional resources responsible for other parts of clinical medicine. Departments, very isolated from each other, were responsible for tuberculosis and for HIV/AIDS even though comorbidities were very common. One of the results of this was the not-infrequent undermanagement of one or the other of the two diseases found together in the same patient.

Russian physicians visiting the United States made some frequent and interesting observations on this matter: "We were surprised that the community is very tolerant of the HIV-positive persons and that there is no discrimination about them," and "The necessity of the complex, team-based organization of the HIV management has been demonstrated very clearly."[8]

The Russian visitors came to appreciate the enormous importance of good laboratory services—measures of numbers of viral particles (viral load) and T-cell lymphocytes (CD4 count)—both for a timely and valid diagnosis and to assist in the ongoing management of the disease.

An area of notable success involved improvement in a clinical program to interrupt mother-to-child transmission of the AIDS virus. Timely recognition of AIDS infection among pregnant mothers prior to giving birth became an opportunity for preventing infection of the newborn. This identification of HIV-positive mothers and treatment with antiretroviral drugs prior to parturition led to a dramatic reduction in infant infection and subsequent HIV disease.

Blagoveshchensk was a particularly interesting story. The city, located on the Amur River directly across from the Chinese city of Hreihe, is a beautiful setting. Blagoveshchensk was a stopping off place for Anton Chekov on his trek to Sakhalin Island in 1890.

A monument to him sits in the city center. A highly entrepreneurial citizen of Balgoveshchensk, Ivan Yakovlevich Churin, pursued a variety of commercial activities in the late nineteenth century between Harbin, Manchuria, and Russia. His mark is everywhere in the city, including a modern Churin Hotel. All of this was in sight of young Russian youths rollerblading along the river's edge with the Chinese shore in the background and Lenin's statue in the foreground.

The medical program was impressive, and the organized discussion with the physician community drew a very large group of participants. The host for this session was the Amur State Medical Academy. The principal spokesman was Dr. Vladimir A. Dorovskih, president of the academy and chairman, Department of Pharmacology.

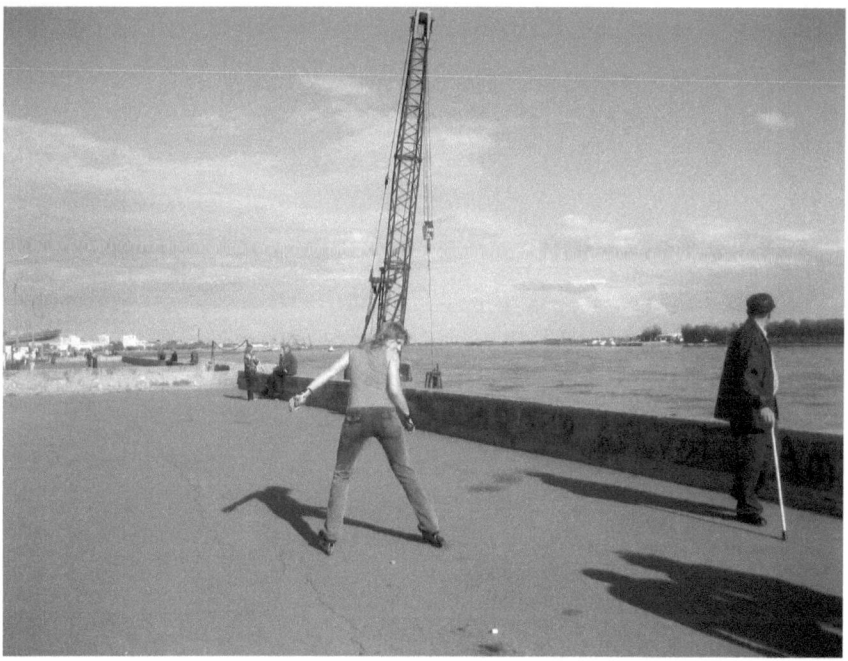

A Scene in Blagoveshchensk

As impressive as this setting was, it was subject to a substantial decline in population numbers in parallel with all of the Russian Far East.

Table 7. Population of Blagoveshchensk and Amur Oblast

	1994	2006
Blagoveshchensk	200,000	90,000
Amur Oblast	1,074,000	881,000

5

The Results: What the Program Accomplished

The nominal goal of the Eurasian Medical Education Program was the enhancement of the capacity of the Russian medical profession to manage serious disease. The commodity we brought to the scene to share with fellow medical professionals was medical scientific information. A second goal, which emerged during the course of the program, was to help reintroduce some of the elements of professionalism that had been lacking for years.

First of all, the program sought to reach and interact with members of the Russian medical profession in a fashion that exercised appropriate leverage. The initial question was, how many of our host physicians did we expose to the elements of the program directly or indirectly? Those attending the continuing medical education sessions over the seventeen-year period of the program in thirteen regions of the Russian Federation numbered well over ten thousand. The didactic materials prepared for the programs reached a larger audience. The visual and printed materials prepared for presentations were always made available for further distribution. The academic medical centers, as we had anticipated, became the vehicle for extending the reach of the program. Importantly, individual sessions of the Eurasian Medical Education Program were frequently scheduled to combine with the Russians' own continuing medical education programs. This allowed the substance of the program to reach groups of practitioners from locations within the academic medical centers, as well as those from more distant settings. Finally, on occasion, the program materials, at the request of the Russian Federation Ministry of Health, were adopted at that level to become part of the fabric of postgraduate medical education broadly.

A next level of assessment undertaken by the program beyond the simple enumeration of attendees was to take the measure of how well the educational materials were understood, how effective the presentations were and how they were received. For this, the program developed two simple instruments: a short questionnaire inquiring after the appropriateness and quality of the presentations, and a short test administered before the lectures and repeated following the sessions. The questions were designed to test the participants' knowledge and determine the extent of understanding and interpretation of the technical medical discussion. Comparison of the results from the pre- and postlecture tests, it was hoped, would provide some indication of the acquisition and understanding of the substantive matters discussed. It also served as a test of the quality of the lectures and the effectiveness of the presentations. This latter instrument was used for a few years early in the program but was eventually discontinued because of objections from our Russian colleagues. An alternative and even better vehicle for this purpose was clinical teaching rounds. The individual sessions almost always included small-group clinical teaching rounds with patients. This traditional teaching device in medicine allowed much discussion and provided an opportunity to take the measure of comprehension of the clinical material of interest. The vast majority of our Russian colleagues participated in these bedside teaching sessions.

The ultimate indication of success of the program, of course, was to be seen in the effective management of underlying disease and the reduction of complications. The desired end point, of course, was a reduction in the burden of disease and mortality.

Improvement in clinical outcomes of disease is seen in cure, remission, decrease in symptoms, decrease in short-term complications, or decrease in the prominence of comorbidities. There are a number of variables linking the continuing medical educational effort to clinical outcomes. Some of these include the translation of educational material into clinical practice; availability of therapeutic tools including drugs in clinical practice; organization of the medical system to foster screening, treatment, and follow-up; and timely medical laboratory resources.

The challenge of identifying and measuring ultimate clinical outcomes for chronic and infectious and noninfectious disease is a substantial one due to long prodromes and latent periods and necessarily long treatment periods to lead to remissions and cures. Thus the program was limited to reliance on proxy measures at the front end of the process. For disease entities, (cardiovascular disease, diabetes, tuberculosis and diabetes) the program established follow-up systems in three regions to track and document patterns of recognition, management, and outcomes of disease. These systems depended on the superb cooperation and technical skills of the departments of epidemiology and statistics in each of the centers. This involved two goals:

- **Alterations in physician practice patterns following the educational sessions.** The aim here was to determine whether patterns of medical practice tended to reflect contemporary standards of care. Measures to observe were the extent to which physicians followed blood pressure or indications of diabetes over time with appropriate therapeutic interventions. Did physicians use laboratory information to monitor TB and HIV treatment, or mother-to-child HIV transmission? Rigorous follow-up depended on systematic review of patient charts over time. We pursued this study with our colleagues for a period limited by the expense of the process.
- **Indices of patient health.** Again, with the cooperation of our colleagues in the individual departments of epidemiology and statistics, the program supported the following of trends of morbidity and mortality, disabilities, and complications.

One other intervention, which strongly influenced health outcomes, was hypertension schools. Russian practitioners, in general, did not devote much time to counseling patients about risk factors' contribution to disease. We adopted a pattern of "schools" designed to serve that purpose for diabetes and cardiovascular disease. From the experience in another Russian seting, Dubna., we developed a pattern of schools concerned with diabetes and hypertension. Subjects included obesity, cigarette smoking, alcohol intake, exercise, and the importance of complying with prescribed drug therapy. For those patients attending the sessions, the importance of prevention of disease and the promotion of health was evident. Unfortunately, as noted earlier, the majority of attendees were relatively elderly women, while the important burden of disease and premature mortality was seen among younger males during their productive years. This was the population that exhibited risky behavior and suffered its consequences.

Examples of Results

Cardiovascular Disease

Overwhelmingly, the major contributor to premature or excess mortality in Russia is cardiovascular disease—myocardial infarction (heart attack) and stroke.

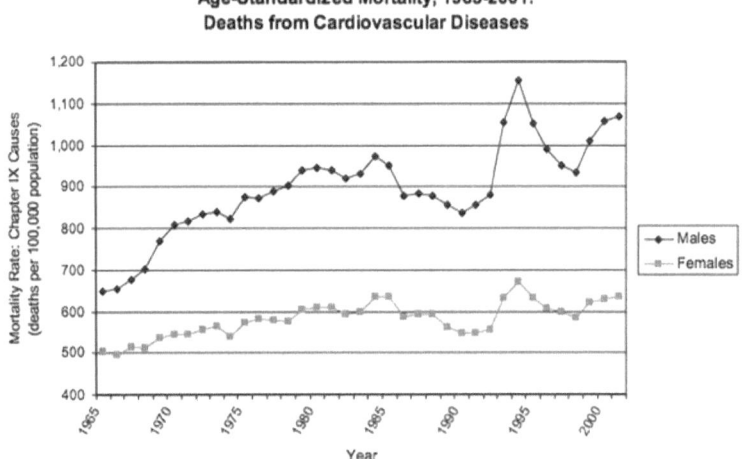

Age-Standardized Mortality, 1965-2001: Deaths from Cardiovascular Diseases

Source: State Committee of the Russian Federation on Statistics, The Demographic Yearbook of Russia: 2002 Statistical Handbook (Moscow: Goskomstat of Russia), 2002.

A principal risk factor for these is elevated blood pressure. This is characteristically a silent process. Patients are typically unaware of hypertension until a serious complication occurs. It has been estimated that only 8% of hypertensives were recognized in Russia, in contrast to over 60% in the United States. Therefore, an appropriate goal of the program was to identify individuals with elevated blood pressure and place them on appropriate pharmacologic and nonpharmacologic therapy.

We inaugurated a program of chronic disease management in hypertension in three regions in Russia: Kazan, Khabarovsk, and Ekaterinburg. The focus in each case was hypertension and the sequelae that followed. Subjects were recruited from those with elevated blood pressure. Patients were screened and followed in polyclinics associated with an academic medical school in each case. All were enrolled initially in a hypertension school.

The cohorts of patients who participated were overwhelmingly females, leading one to speculate that the middle-aged, employed Russian male was a truly endangered species. In Khabarovsk, we followed a group of 869 patients for three years. In this cohort:

- Hypertension control increased by 49%.
- Absenteesim from the workplace setting due to illness decreased by 73%.
- Average residence in hospital decreased by 76%.
- For those patients who were hospitalized, length of stay decreased by 47%.

The hypertension program in Ekaterinburg revealed similar results. Again, among those who were followed, 34% were males and 65% were females. Seventy-five to eighty percent of the patients showed left ventricular hypertrophy (thickening of the walls of the ventricles of the heart). This was evidence of the chronicity of the disease and was the first evidence of end-organ impact of elevated blood pressure. As many as 14% of patients already had a history of myocardial infarction (heart attack), and 9.4% reported a history of stroke. Eighty-five percent of the patients were overweight, and elevated blood lipids were found in 50%. However, the stage of hypertension damage still indicated that the patients could benefit from chronic, persistent, and effective therapy.

The disease management program in Ekaterinburg demonstrated the following results at the end of three months:

- Blood pressure was reduced in 46%.
- Blood cholesterol was reduced in 33%.
- There was a marked increase in compliance with medications and nonpharmacologic therapy.
- Smoking was reduced.

Diabetes

Uniquely, diabetic patients in Russia who are registered with the government receive regular supervision and free medication. A consequence of this is a near 100% recognition of patients with diabetes. In cooperation with our colleagues, we followed and managed large cohorts of diabetic patients over three years in Khabarovsk and one a one-half years in Kazan.

In Khabarovsk (7,211 patients), at the end of two years:

- Diabetic complications were reduced.
- Incidence of ketoacidosis (abnormal metabolic consequence of inadequate or insufficient presence of insulin) was reduced.
- Incidence of diabetic foot syndrome (a consequence of diabetic neuropathy, traumatic injury, and compromised healing) was reduced.
- Gangrene as a cause of death was reduced by 71% relative to an earlier baseline incidence.

In Ekaterinburg, the program followed 16,200 patients for three years with the following results:

- Diabetic complications were reduced
- Ketoacidosis was reduced by 38%.
- Diabetic foot syndrome was reduced by 19%.

In Kazan, we followed 353 patients for eighteen months with the following results:

- Hospital treatment for diabetic complications decreased by 35%.
- Adherence to diabetic diet improved.
- Attendance at diabetic schools increased by 34%.

Tuberculosis

At the beginning of the Eurasian Medical Education Program, Russia was heavily burdened by tuberculosis infection and complications and by tuberculosis mortality. The incidence of TB and tuberculosis mortality fell in Russia until the early 1990s, when TB mortality, especially among males, began to rise precipitously (see figure).

Traditionally, tuberculosis infection and as a cause of death were thought of as affecting the elderly. The reasons, long recognized, included crowding, impoverishment, and social disorganization. An additional factor in Russia was the rise of HIV/AIDS. In Russia, TB joined other chronic diseases such as cardiovascular disease and diabetes as a cause of morbidity and premature mortality among young and middle-aged individuals—especially males in their most productive years.

In the early 1990s, with the breakup of the Soviet system, the formerly effective public health system also disintegrated. There was an insufficiency of therapeutic drugs to treat the disease. The incidence of TB in prisons and among those discharged or amnestied from prison was exceedingly high. Discharged prisoners (around three hundred thousand a year) were released into civilian neighborhoods with little or no follow-up, representing a prominent source of new infection. It was estimated that 10%, or thirty thousand, released prisoners exhibited active TB, and 25% of those had multidrug-resistant TB (MDRTB).

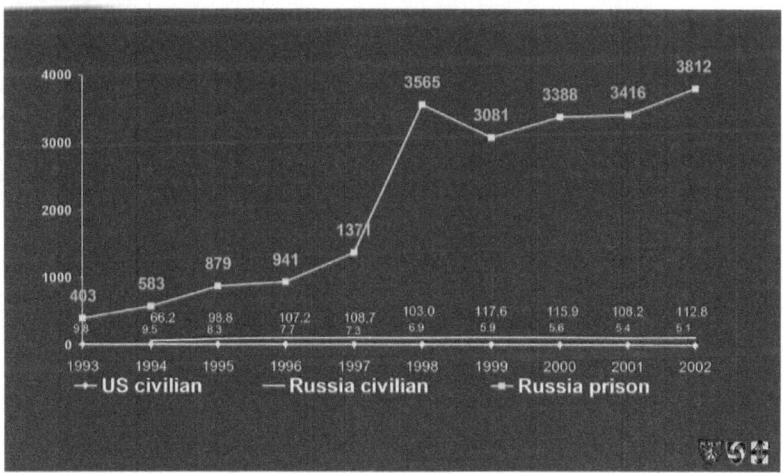

Figure 4. TB case notification (incidence) per 100,000 population, 1993–2002

The principal causes of the high level of MDRTB and XDRTB in Russia were delayed diagnosis and inadequate or inappropriate therapy leading to primary drug resistance.

Importantly, the traditional pattern of management of tuberculosis in Russia stood in the way of successful resolution of the TB epidemic:

- Rather than adhering to a recognized standard set of protocols for TB, Russian medical practice favored "individualized" treatment. Prikaz (order) number 33, the basic law governing physician behavior, permitted physicians to exercise individual, professional judgment rather than an accepted standard of care in treating the disease.
- Controversies over reliance on surgery and tuberculosis have already been mentioned. Russian medical practice relied on surgery for tuberculosis, resulting in the controversies discussed earlier.
- There was heavy reliance in Russia on prolonged inpatient care. All patients had to be hospitalized for a period of at least eight weeks. Western patterns of care for drug-sensitive disease included an initial three days of outpatient care. The reasons for this reliance on inpatient management became clear early. In Russia, there are 334,000 pulmonary hospital beds and 10,000 lung physicians. The pay of the hard-pressed medical staff was based on the number of filled hospital beds and the number of surgical procedures completed. A switch to a regime requiring personnel with fewer qualifications to administer drugs to patients living at home or seen in dispensary settings meant the redeployment or unemployment of many.

Patient compliance with medication was recognized early as a problem in dealing with tuberculosis. Interruption in treatment was an acknowledged factor contributing to drug-resistant disease. The Russian response to this problem was enforced inpatient (and therefore observed) administration of drugs. The World Health Organization recommended the DOTS (Direct observation therapy short course) pattern of drug for ambulatory patients where the patient is observed while taking where the patient is observed while taking schedule drugs. This is combined with incentives to encourage compliance. The DOTS pattern in outpatient settings was fiercely resisted initially in Russia as it threatened the tradition of inpatient care.

What emerged as a principal problem in Russian settings was a lack of effective and timely laboratory resources and systems to establish accurate diagnoses and determine the sensitivity of organisms from lung specimens. The results of diagnostic investigations were typically reported after a delay of three months rather than a required four to five weeks. Further, in many cases, characterization of the pathologic organisms was performed not by microbiological tests, but by methods of molecular biology that were incapable of determining drug sensitivity. This resulted in treating physicians prescribing drugs without knowledge of sensitivity—the major cause of drug-resistant disease. As one of our visiting experts observed, "Overall, we found the TB laboratory operations the weakest part of future efforts to control tuberculosis."

The Eurasian Medical Education Program concentrated its efforts in tuberculosis in regions exhibiting a high burden of disease and which were known for outstanding technical skill. Ekaterinburg, Khabarovsk, Birobidzhan, Irkutsk, and Novosibirsk were key examples. The program mounted multiple visits to each of these and also brought delegations of Russian TB specialists, laboratory specialists, and health workers to New Jersey Medical Center and the National Jewish Medical and Research Center. These were the outstanding centers for tuberculosis in the United States. Visiting physicians typically spent a month in residence, steeped in clinical work, the DOTS pattern of treatment, and laboratory techniques. These sessions ultimately proved to be very effective. Acceptance and adoption generally required a few years, as the main principles ran counter to established Russian practice and were contrary to the existing rules promulgated by the Russian Federation Ministry of Health.

It was apparent early that the task of influencing tuberculosis control in Russia was a complex one. The legacy of long-entrenched medical tradition and bureaucratic constraint made for a substantial challenge. The program that evolved focused on five components:

- **Effective case finding for new cases of tuberculosis infection and active tuberculosis.** An important goal was recognition of drug-resistant disease. The Russian system relied heavily on chest x-ray for diagnosis. Radiological diagnosis lacked specificity, and interpretation could be confused by other nontuberculosis conditions. What was clearly needed was a strong diagnostic laboratory system, based on biological principles (culture and sensitivity), which could deliver specific diagnostic results within a short period of time. Because of the importance of the diagnostic laboratory, we developed a detailed plan for appropriate laboratory services, entitled "Ural Model of the TB Laboratory Support System as Part of the Comprehensive TB Control Program."[1] The plan was called the Ural Model because it was first developed for the Sverdlovsk Region but it was generally applicable throughout Russia. The plan offered detailed recommendations concerning equipment and culture techniques. It proposed a centralized laboratory and included a program for rapid reporting of results.
- **Effective treatment based on culture-proven diagnosis.** Effective therapy implied standardized therapy for drug-sensitive disease. From experience elsewhere in the world, standardized therapy meant three first-line drugs without interruption for six months.
- **Assurance of compliance with therapy.** A compromise was made with our Russian colleagues to provide for an initial inpatient oversight of TB therapy followed by a longer period of observed ambulatory care—a modified form of direct observation therapy.
- **High priority for TB control programs.** Highest priority was given to the identification and treatment of drug-sensitive individuals. At the same time, the need for additional support was recognized for drug-resistant cases.
- **Special attention to the issues of tuberculosis in prisons.** The jurisdiction for this was the Russian Federation Ministry of Justice. Prevalence of tuberculosis and drug-resistant tuberculosis was exceedingly high among prisoners and those subject to short-term detention. TB was commonly admixed with other comorbidities, particularly HIV/AIDS. As noted earlier, an im-

portant issue was the release of approximately three hundred thousand prisoners per year into the community without any follow-up. This represented a constant "pump" or source of more disease into the general population.

HIV/AIDS

The first reported case of HIV infection in Russia was in October 1985. An explosive increase in incidence and prevalence became evident in the years 1996 to 1997. One thousand new cases were registered in 1995. That increased to 250,000 new cases in 2002.

This period, encompassing the last of the former Soviet Union and the early days of the Russian Federation, was marked by an extraordinary pattern of forces—social, political, governmental, professional, and economic—arrayed against an accurate accounting of the epidemic and, hence, its proper management.

The disease was officially and socially denied. Principal risk groups—prostitutes and narcotic drug users—were denied or subject to legal sanction[2] Stigma and discrimination marked the medical profession generally. Isolation of the Russian population from knowledge about the problem, combined with frank disinformation, severely reduced preventive and corrective action. Scapegoating was prominent. The Soviets had claimed that AIDS had been manufactured by the U.S. Centers for Disease Control and Prevention (CDC) and the Pentagon.[3] Nevertheless, the Soviet government took initial steps to provide a legal basis for testing and prevention in a law passed in 1987. Unfortunately, it focused heavily on punitive measures.

Murray Feshbach pointed to an astounding letter written by a group of sixteen young medical graduates to the director of the Central Epidemiological Research Institute in 1987:

> Dear Colleagues: We graduates of a medical institution are categorically opposed to combating the new "disease" AIDS! And we intend to do everything in our power to impede the search for ways to combat that noble epidemic. We are convinced that within a short time AIDS will destroy all drug addicts and prostitutes. We are confident that Hippocrates would have approved of our decision. Long live AIDS![4]

Substantial uncertainty surrounded the true size of the burden of HIV infection and AIDS as a disease. In 2007, UNAIDS estimated the prevalence of HIV to be between 850,000 and 1,000,000. The U.S. National Intelligence Council in 2002 predicted a prevalence of three to four million cases by 2010.[5]

Several prominent risk groups and patterns of risky behavior were identified. These included heterosexual transmission, homosexual transmission, contamination of blood supply, and unprotected sex. Overwhelmingly, the most prominent risk group for HIV/AIDS leading to the explosive epidemic was intravenous drug use and contaminated syringes in the late 1990s during the momentous political transition.

During this period, the medical profession was unprepared to respond to the AIDS challenge and was not appropriately supported to confront the task. Diagnostic techniques were not universally recognized. Antiviral drugs were in short supply. AIDS clinics and departments were isolated from other specialty groups. Until the 2000s, the Russian government response was one of awkward silence. HIV/AIDS was not a priority. In the early 2000s, the Russian government gradually began to shift its position from denial and neglect to one of active interest and participation. In his 2003 speech to the nation, President Putin mentioned HIV/AIDS publicly. In 2005, the president announced a dramatic increase in the budget dedicated to HIV/AIDS, which rose from $150 million in 2006 to $300 million in 2007. A governmental commission on AIDS was established in 2006 and met for the first time in January 2007. Simultaneously, five Russian nongovernmental organizations made a successful application to the Global Fund. This embarrassed the Russian government into further action and brought forth a grant of $270 million for the AIDS challenge.

The majority of this money was devoted to therapeutic drugs. It became apparent that with a new and augmented source of therapeutic agents, the profession lacked standards of care and knowledge about the management of the disease. Academic medical centers did proceed to establish departments devoted to HIV/AIDS, albeit separated from other clinical specialty groups. Infectious disease specialists identified themselves as devoted to a specialty concerned with AIDS.

The Eurasian Medical Education Program focused on HIV/AIDS in March 2007 in Ekaterinburg. This was followed by eleven subsequent missions to Russian centers in eight regions of the Russian Federation. These missions were combined with visits of Russian AIDS specialists to institutions in the United States. The program shared with large groups of Russian infectious disease specialists the extensive experience of management of HIV/AIDS as it had evolved in other parts of the world. Sessions lasting over several days included:

- Biological details of the AIDS virus and its interaction with immune defense mechanisms, which provided the biological mechanistic basis for drug treatment
- Evaluation and use of antiretroviral agents, which by this time had grown from one to nineteen
- Highly active antiretroviral therapy for resistant organisms
- Coinfection and opportunistic infections, with particular attention given to tuberculosis (Approximately one-half of deaths of AIDS patients are due to TB.)
- The role of the laboratory for diagnosing and monitoring HIV infection and for monitoring therapy Management of HIV for special groups—children, women, pregnancy
- The extremely important role of adherence to therapy without interruption

Concern for Professionalism

Alongside the principal focus of the program concerned with clinical management of disease, we found a second opportunity for constructive interaction. Soviet physicians were restricted in their ability to travel to professional meetings and engage in a variety of ways collectively recognized as elements of professional association and professionalism. We found an understandable hunger to reestablish these elements of professionalism. Our hosts constantly sought opportunities for collaboration in clinical research and for professional publication.

In modest fashion, we were able to arrange for opportunities in both cases. The work in cardiovascular disease became the subject of several professional publications with joint authorship. We fostered several collaborative epidemiological investigations designed to examine the effectiveness of screening and management of vascular hypertension in relation to serious cardiovascular events and complications. We examined together a series of questions relating to the Russian heavy dependence on BCG vaccine use and subsequent reported pathological complications in bone disease. We participated in a large number of medical-scientific seminars and named lectures. From this came published papers in both American and Russian medical journals.

6

Health: An Instrument of Engagement

As stated at the beginning of this work, the nominal goal of the Eurasian Medical Education Program was to share contemporary understanding of the pathophysiology of disease with Russian practitioners and to provide current standards of care. It was hoped that this would enhance the capacity of the medical profession in Russia to manage serious disease. For this, we chose a traditional educational vehicle, recognized throughout the world of medicine: continuing medical education. As we anticipated, this turned out to be an excellent choice. It assured a high professional level of interaction and preserved professional respect for both parties. Since the Russian medical profession had a tradition of its own of obligatory continuing medical education, into which we fit our sessions, the arrangement facilitated the sharing of clinical experience in both directions. That is, our visiting experts were able to learn of Russian experience and patterns of care.

But there was a further and important goal of the program. As director, I was keenly interested in the larger political framework in which the program operated. The questions here were: How did the program fit into or articulate with U.S.-Russian relations? To what extent did it interact with or complement U.S. foreign policy goals?

The thesis expressed in this work is that, in our relations with Russia, engagement rather than isolation is in the interests of both parties.[1] The several-decades-long period since the end of the Soviet Union has been marked by periods of both active efforts at engagement and cooperation, and periods when engagement was explicitly discouraged on both sides. These cycles were in part the result of external forces acting on the two nations and in part a function of deep-seated cultural differences. Initial enthusiasm in the early 1990s was replaced by 1999 during the severe economic crisis in Russia with disaffection with promises made of a better life under a market economy. The 1990s were perceived by many in Russia as a period of vulnerability and one where America policies were designed to take advantage of or perpetuate Russian weakness. This was in sharp contrast to a central Russian objective of regaining its stature as a great power commanding respect parallel to that of the United States.

There exists a substantial body of academic work concerned with health and foreign policy.[2] There is a long history of foreign-directed efforts explicitly dedicated to containing health threats that exhibit the potential of crossing international boundaries. The threat of cholera brought states together to coordinate quarantine efforts 150 years ago. Yellow fever was a matter of international common concern at the time of the building of the Panama Canal.

There is a similarly long history of international cooperation and coordination of efforts aimed at containing or even eradicating the pathogenic organisms recognized responsible for serious and life-threatening disease—smallpox and poliomyelitis. Foreign policy attention to these matters has received increasing visibility in recent years, in part because of an increase in potential hazards from natural outbreaks and epidemics and, in part because of threats from human-directed attempts to use microbiological agents as weapons.[3] All of these may be categorized as foreign policy responses to security-related health threats.

A different aspect of health in relation to foreign policy is captured by the phrase "health as an instrument of foreign policy." Implied here is the explicit concentration on health abroad as a foreign policy goal or as a means to achieve a particular security or foreign policy goal. The Marshall Plan was propelled by both charitable and security concerns. Economic and social dislocation threatened western Europe following World War II. Ill health and poverty were prominent, and the Marshall Plan included elements designed to address those challenges.[4]

One of the most successful examples was a fifteen-year cooperative health program in Latin America in the early 1940s with both security and social and economic development as goals. World War II was on the horizon. Motivation for this initiative was a combination of humanitarian interests and security concerns. Forward planning for the anticipated conflict recognized the importance of Brazil as a desired location for staging troops on their way to North Africa. To use this location required the eradication of malaria. Additionally, the United States desired a source of natural resources (rubber) and wished to reduce the Nazi influence present in Argentina. In 1942, Nelson Rockefeller, impressed with the importance of health as a vital element in Latin American social and economic development, and with the strong support of President Roosevelt, established a quasigovernmental corporation, the Institute for Inter-American Affairs, devoted to health and medicine assistance for eighteen Latin American nations. The extragovernmental form was chosen explicitly to allow for flexibility, to encourage contributions by professionals from the academic and foundation communities (especially the Rockefeller Foundation), and to avoid the burdensome restrictions of normal U.S. governmental regulations. The United States committed itself to a long-term project with a set level of funding. The understanding in all cases was that the host Latin American country would eventually assume 100% of the cost.

The program was extremely successful. From the beginning, it worked closely with host governments. It enjoyed a substantial continuity and longevity, coming to an end only in 1958. The program, in collaboration with the Rockefeller Foundation, built hospitals, nursing schools, and health clinics and supported training programs for visiting nurses and health education programs for the general public. Among its most important characteristics were coherence of effort, the continuity of long-term dedication, a strong element of professionalism, and a sense of partnership and cooperation rather than a donor-recipient relationship.[5] The principles so important in this successful example were unfortunately forgotten and not repeated at any time subsequently. In 1948, borrowing on the experience in Latin America, a more modest effort of similar character was put in place as part of the Point Four Program in Greece.[6]

Health as an Instrument of Engagement

Underlying the concentration on health is a desire to reduce the probability of social and political unrest. Much has been written about the aspects of poverty and ill health as environments ripe for or fostering social unrest and conflict.[7] Focus on health in this sense recognizes the importance of human capital and the importance of giving value to existing human capital. These are understood as imperatives for pursuing social and political stability and preventing conflict.[8]

The United States had a self-interest in seeking opportunities for engagement in the health sector in Russia. Excess or premature mortality contributed prominently to the now well-recognized demographic decline. Negative consequences of these trends were recognized for both security and economic security with consequences for social order.[9] A Congressional report written in 2000 commented at length on U.S.-Russia relations. While a highly partisan document in many ways, its constructive and statesman-like conclusions emphasized the interest of the United States and the West in a stable and secure Russian nation able to exercise its economic potential as a trading partner. The recommendations of that report were surprising, considering the origin of the report. Among them was one that remains valid: "The United States, our friends and allies, and the world are more threatened today by Russian economic, political and social weaknesses than by Russian strength."[10]

This was also the message of the 2007 report, "CSIS Commission on Smart Power," from the Center for Strategic and International Studies.[11] That report singled out health as a special opportunity for engagement. Biomedical science served as the currency for engagement with the Soviet Union in 1972 during the period of detente.[12] The program concerned with cardiovascular and pulmonary disease in cooperation with the cardiology center in Moscow, devoted to scientific exchanges, spanned a period exceeding thirty years.[13]

The seventeen-year period of the Eurasian Medical Education Program in Russia was one marked by remarkable and dynamic changes and turmoil in U.S.-Russian relationships. The relationships moved from euphoria to disappointment several times during the period. The Eurasian Medical Education Program began its activities in 1995. By1998, with severe devaluation of the Russian ruble, the economy was in serious trouble. Important was the nearly exclusive dependence on extractive resources and the absence of any serious effort to diversify the economy.[14] This eventually became a serious political and social issue when the GDP fell by 3.5% in 2005 and inflation rose to 15%, threatening the ability of the government to pay pensions.[15]

Duma elections of 2012 led to street demonstrations blamed officially on "outside forces." The Russian leadership was increasingly unhappy over the failure of acceptance of Russia as a major world power. The Kremlin faced a series of threats from the Republic of Chechnya, leading ultimately to two formal Chechen wars. Russian ventures in the Republic of Georgia and later in Ukraine were symptomatic of an increasingly unhappy and presumably insecure Russian leadership. The leadership repeatedly complained about U.S.-related actions seemingly unfriendly to Russia. Among the prominent examples were NATO enlargement eastward following the reunification of Germany, U.S. unilateral revoking of the 1972 Anti-Ballistic Missile Treaty, and a threatened establishment of a missile defense system within the borders of former Warsaw pact neighbors.

Throughout this turbulent period, the Eurasian Medical Education Program continued an uninterrupted and active course of engagement with Russia. The experience of the Eurasian Medical Education Program was immune to any adverse or diverting political influence.

Throughout this tumultuous period the Eurasian Medical Education Progam proceeded without interruption. More than that, in fact the program expanded from an original five regions of the Russian Federation to thirteen, stretching across nearly all of the eleven time zones of the Russian land mass. Our Russian colleagues consistently encouraged us to expand and extend our activities both in substance and geographically. The leadership of two of the regions offered assistance in financial support for the program.

The purpose of this chapter is to assert that engagement with, not isolation from, Russia was in the interest of both parties. Former Russian statesmen have argued that Russia must avoid "self-isolation...and keep the door open to cooperation with the U.S. and its allies in the North Atlantic Treaty Organization. Former prime minister and foreign minister Yevgeny Primakov declared that "we close our country in a great power without such collaboration." Former finance minister, Alexei Kudrin, stated that Russia faces a "full-fledged economic crisis if it doesn't repair its ties with the U.S. and Europe

Referring again to the Congressional report written in 2000 cited earlier, social and economic order in Russia remain in the interest of the United States. Clearly, the fact that both countries share 95% of the nuclear weapons is a persuasive argument. To fail to build lines of communication and cooperation threatens a prospect of a very unpredictable Russian leadership.

The experience of the Eurasian Medical Education Program proved again that health is an excellent instrument for engagement. The program reached well over ten thousand physicians in Russia during the course of seventeen years. It relied on the offices of the political and medical leadership in thirteen regions of the federation. Our contributing American physician experts were given faculty recognition in several instances. Several of us were invited to take active roles in important named lecture series and celebrations. As director, I was elected a corresponding member of the Russian Academy of Medical Sciences. Finally, all of this occurred at a time of substantial political turmoil in Russia and marked shifts in official U.S.-Russian relationships.

Epilogue

We began the Eurasian Medical Education Program as an experiment. The primary goal was to craft an effort that was likely to make a tangible and, perhaps, important contribution to the medical sector in Russia. In the view of this author, we succeeded in that desire at three levels. The first was to enhance the capacity of practitioners to manage serious disease by sharing experience and knowledge as the basis of contemporary standards of care. The second was to collaborate in recapturing traditional elements of professionalism. Both of these goals were considered appropriate following the seventy years of relative isolation of the Russian medical system.

The program eventually took on a much larger scale than first conceived. To a great extent, this was a reflection of an invitation for ever more and more frequent actions invited by our colleagues in Russia. In fact, the frequency of our efforts was limited only by the financial resources available.

At least as important was the contribution the program made to engage Russia. This was borne out dramatically by the reception the program received even during the periods of heightened political tension.

There were elements of the program that were clearly important for its success:

- Our partnership with the American College of Physicians was of enormous importance. The American College of Physicians brought with it outstanding physician resources and instructive materials that were highly respected abroad. This pattern stood in stark contrast to the majority of "foreign assistance" efforts managed by contractors for the U.S. government.

- The visiting physician experts were specifically chosen from among those whose own professional contributions were substantial and recognized. In this way, they were viewed as peers by our colleagues abroad.
- We religiously avoided any sense of "training." Rather, the spirit was that of *sharing* experience and knowledge in both directions.
- Continuity of the effort over time emerged as highly important. There was a universe of unknown size of well-meaning church groups, hospitals, and individuals who traveled to Russian centers one time only. Our hosts, clearly weary of that pattern, urged a sustaining relationship with strong professional ties.
- Our strategy of centering efforts on the thirteen regions of the Russian Federation rather than on the major population centers of Moscow and St. Petersburg turned out to be a key decision.
- Financial support for the program was approximately one-half from nongovernmental sources. This was essential in preserving the professional character of the program and went far in isolating the programmatic decisions from frequent U.S. government political changes.

In September 2012, the Russian Ministry of Foreign Affairs declared that institutions supported by the U.S. Agency for International Development were no longer welcome in Russia. The Kremlin's increasing unhappiness with political influence of human rights and promotion of democracy emerged as the background of the announcement; health and medicine were not part of that background. We ascertained this from a trip to Moscow in 2013 in the company of one of our former ambassadors to Russia. The trip included a series of meetings with senior officials in the Russian Ministry of Foreign Affairs, as well as others. The meetings were designed to examine two questions: Is there still an appetite for cooperation in the health sector, and if so, might there be a source of Russian funds to help support the program? The responses to both questions were in the affirmative. Unfortunately, by this time there were no sources of financial support from the U.S. side. Hostility toward Russia among members of the American public was intense. The posture of the State Department and the National Security Council was to isolate and avoid Russia.

A final event occurred related to the program. The background is a respected institution in Oxford, England, known as the Cochrane Collaboration. The Cochrane Collaboration had been established in 1993 to review the quality and the validity of the evidentiary basis for medical procedures and interventions. The Cochrane Collaboration has become the reference point fofr that judgment. In 2015, the Cochrane Collaboration elected to establish a Cochrane Russia institution to further its goal. It chose the Kazan State Medical University as its locus and our colleague there as the director. In December 2015 the Cochrane institution in Kazan was opened, and I was asked to assist in opening that new center. The significance of this event is particularly interesting. The appointment of the academic medical center in Russia, after seven decades of isolation, represented a large measure of support for the medical leadership. It was a well-deserved honor.

Notes

Chapter 1

1. Mark G. Field, "Medicine in the Context of Russian History and Culture: An American Perspective" (paper presented at the International Conference on the Education of Family Physicians and Lessons for America and the World, National Institutes of Health, Washington, D.C., October 26–29, 1995).
2. Nicholas V. Riasanovsky, *A History of Russia* (New York: Oxford University Press, 2000).
3. See note 1 above.
4. See note 1 above.
5. Diane Rowland and Alexandre V. Telyukov, "Soviet Health Care from Two Perspectives," *Health Affairs* 10, no. 2 (1991): 71–86
6. William A. Knaus, *Inside Russian Medicine: An American Doctor's First-Hand Report* (Boston: Everest House Publishers, 1981).
7. Mark G. Field, "Medical Care in the Soviet Union," in *The Quality of Life in the Soviet Union*, ed. Horst Herlemann (Boulder, CO: Westview Press, 1987).
8. Mark G. Field, "Medical Care in the Soviet Union: Promises and Realities" (paper presented at conference, The Quality of Life in the Soviet Union, Kennan Institute for Advanced Russian Studies, Washington, D.C., August 1, 1984).
9. Sarah Helmstadter, "Medical Insurance in Russia," *RFE/RL Research Report* 1, no. 32 (July 31, 1992): 65–69.
10. Mark G. Field, "Post-Communist Medicine: Morbidity, Mortality and the Deteriorating Health Situation" (paper presented at conference, The Social Legacy of Communism, Institute of Sino-Soviet Studies, George Washington University, Washington, D.C., February 20–22, 1992).
11. Vladimir M. Shkolnikov, France Meslé, and Jacques Vallin, "Recent Trends in Life Expectancy and Causes of Death in Russia, 1970–1993," in *Premature Death in the New Independent States*, ed. José Luis Bobadilla, Christine A. Costello, and Faith Mitchell (Washington, D.C.: National Academy Press, 1997), 61–65.

12. Ibid.
13. Sergei A. Vassin and Christine A. Costello, Faith Mitchell (Washington, D.C.: National Academy Press, 1997).
14. See note 11 above.
15. Mark G. Field, "The Health and Demographic Crisis in Post-Soviet Russia: A Two-Phase Development," in *Russia's Torn Safety Nets: Health and Social Welfare During the Transition*, ed. Mark G. Field and Judyth L. Twigg (New York: St. Martin's Press, 2000), 11–42;and Mark G. Field, "The Health Crisis in the Former Soviet Union: A Report from the 'Post-War Zone,'" *Social Science & Medicine* 41, no. 11 (December 1995): 1469-78.

Chapter 2

1. Jeffrey Sachs and P. Boone, "Strengthening Western Support for Russia's Economic Reforms" (unpublished memorandum, December 28, 1992).
2. Graham Allison and Robert D. Blackwill Robert D. Blackwill, " On With the Grand Bargain," *Washington Post*, August 27, 1991.
3. Nicholas V. Riasanovsky, *History of Russia*. (See chap.1, n. 2)
4. Stephen F. Cohen, "U.S. Policy Toward Post-Communist Russia: Fallacies, Failures, Real Possibilities" (testimony before the Committee on Foreign Affairs, U.S. House of Representatives, February 24, 1993).
5. World Bank, "A Marshall Plan Type Technical Assistance Program for the Former Soviet Union" (unpublished memorandum to Russell Cheetham, World Bank, Washington, D.C., November 10, 1992); and Charles J. Weiss, Jack M. Seymour, Charles M. Grohs and Courtney M. Brooks, *The Marshall Plan: Lessons for U.S. Assistance to Central and Eastern Europe and the Former Soviet Union* (Washington, D.C.: The Atlantic Council, December 1995).
6. World Bank, "A Marshall Plan Type Technical Assistance Program." (see note 5 above) 7.
7. Weiss, et al., The Marshall Plan (see note 5 above); Curt Tarnoff, *The Marshall Plan: Design, Accomplishments, and Relevance to the Present* (Washington, D.C.: Congressional Research Service Report, Library of Congress, January 6, 1997), and Lincoln Gordon, "The Marshall Plan and the Former Soviet Union" (paper presented at the symposium Lessons from the Era of the Marshall Plan, Harvard University, Cambridge, MA, June 4, 1997).
8. Lincoln Gordon, "Tasks for a Non-Cold War Era" (paper presented at the Conference on Conflict Prevention and Regional Security into the 21st Century, George C. Marshall European Center for Security Studies, Garmisch-Partenkirchen, Germany, April 27–29, 1997).

9. Medical Working Group, Experts Delegation to the Newly Independent States, conducted February 26–March 31, 1992 for the Coordinating Conference on Assistance to the New Independent States, Lisbon, May 23–24, 1992.
10. Ibid
11. U.S. Agency for International Development, Request for Proposal (RFP) OP/CC/N-93-16, "Health Care Finance and Service Delivery Reform Project No. 110-0004," Washington, D.C., August 4, 1993.
12. Peter J. Stavrakis, "Bull in a China Shop: USAID's Post-Soviet Mission," *Demokratizatsiya*, 4, no. 21 (Spring 1996): 247–70.
13. Dov Chernichovsky, "A Right to Health Insurance Versus a Right to Health Care" (unpublished memorandum, World Bank, Washington, D.C., September 24, 1992).
14. Curt Tarnoff, *The Former Soviet Union and U.S. Foreign Aid: Implementing the Assistance Program* (Washington, D.C.: Congressional Research Service Report, Library of Congress, January 18, 1995).
15. Field, "Health and Demographic Crisis" (see chap.1, n. 15).
16. John Odling-Smee, "The IMF and Russia in the 1990s" (working paper WP/04/155, International Monetary Fund, Washington, D.C., August 2004); Michel Camdessus, "The Transformation of the Russian Economy: Progress Made, Challenges Remaining, and the Role of the IMF" (address presented at Moscow Finance Academy, Moscow, March 21, 1994); Michel Camdessus, "Economic Transformation in the Fifteen Republics of the Former USSR: A Challenge or an Opportunity for the World?" (address presented at Georgetown University School of Foreign Service, Washington, D.C., April 15, 1992); and Michel Camdessus, (address presented at Moscow Institute of International Affairs, Moscow, April 2, 1997).
17. Adam N. Stulberg, *Russia: Facing the Future. A Report of the Carnegie Corporation of New York* (New York: Carnegie Corporation of New York, 2001).
18. Ibid.
19. Charles Krauthammer, "It's *Their* Economy, Stupid," *Washington Post*, February 9, 1996.

Chapter 4

1. Institute of Medicine, *Promoting Cardiovascular Health in the Developing World: A Critical Challenge to Achieve Global Health*, ed. Valentin Fuster and Bfridget B. Kelly (Washington, D.C.: National Academy Press, 2010), Richard Horton, "The Neglected Epidemic of Chronic Disease," *The Lancet* 366, no. 9496 (October 2005), 1514; and World Health

Organization, *Preventing Chronic Diseases: A Vital Investment* (Geneva: World Health Organization, 2005).
2. Stephen Leeder, Susan Raymond, Henry Greenberg, Hui Liu and Kathy Esson, *A Race Against Time*, New York, The Earth Institute at Columbia University and Columbia University Mailman School of Public Health, The University of Sidney and the Center for Global Health and Economic Development, 2004.
3. Erkki Vartiainen, Tiina Laatikainen, Markku Peltonen, Anne Juolevi, Satu Männistö, Jouko Sundvall, Pekka Jousilahti, Veikko Salomaa, Liisa Valsta andPekka Puska, "Thirty-Five-Year Trends in Cardiovascular Risk Factors in Finland," *International Journal of Epidemiology* 39, no. 2 (2010): 504–18.
4. Henry M. Greenberg, Albert S. Galyavich, Lilia E. Ziganshina, Maria R. Tinchurina, Albert G. Chamidullin, and Richard G. Farmer, "Identification and Management of Patients with Hypertension in the Polyclinic System of the Russian Federation," *American Journal of Hypertension* 18 no.7 (2005): 943–48.
5. National Intelligence Council, *The Next Wave of HIV/AIDS: Nigeria, Ethiopia, Russia, India, and China* (Washington, D.C.: National Intelligence Council, ICA 2002-04D, September 2002).
6. C. Rühl, V. Polrovsky, and V. Vinogradov, *The Economic Consequences of HIV in Russia* (Moscow: World Bank, 2002).
7. Kate Dolan, Ben Kite, Emma Black, Carmen Aceijas, and Gerry V. Stimson, "HIV in Prison in Low-Income and Middle-Income Countries," *The Lancet Infectious Diseases* 7, no. 1 (2007): 32–41.
8. Comments to author from AIDS physicians from Yekaterinburg visiting AIDS clinics at Johns Hopkins University, Baltimore, Maryland, March 15, 2004.

Chapter 5

1. L. Heifets, M. Krabchenko, M. Zueva, E. Karelina, and A. Kornienko, "Ural Model of the TB Laboratory Support System as a Part of the Comprehensive TB Control Program" (plan developed for the Eurasian Medical Education Program, National Jewish Medical and Research Center, Denver, Colorado, 2002).
2. Judyth Twigg, *HIV/AIDS in Russia: Commitment, Resources, Momentum, Challenges* (Washington, D.C.: Center for Strategic and International Studies, 2007).
3. Murray Feshbach, "The Early Days of the HIV/AIDS Epidemic in the Former Soviet Union" (paper presented at a conference on Health and Demography in the Former Soviet Union, Harvard University, Cambridge, Massachusetts, April 2005).

4. Ibid
5. National Intelligence Council, *The Next Wave* (see chap. 4, n. 5).

Chapter 6

1. Edward J. Burger and E. Wayne Merry, "Engagement with Russia—Not Isolation—in the Health Sector," *Eurohealth* 14, no. 4 (2009): 25–29.
2. David P. Fidler, "Health and Foreign Policy: A Conceptual Overview" (lecture presented at conference on Health in Foreign Policy Forum, sponsored by Academy Health, Washington, D.C., February 4, 2005) and Ronald Labonté and Michelle L. Gagnon, "Framing Health and Foreign Policy: Lessons for Global Health Diplomacy," *Globalization and Health* 6, no. 14 (2010): 1–19.
3. Rebecca Katz and Daniel A. Singer, "Health and Security in Foreign Policy," *Bulletin of the World Health Organization* 85, no. 3 (March 2007): 233–34.
4. Marcus Schaper, "Health as Foreign Policy: A U.S.-German Dialogue on Governance and Global Health," (paper presented at conference on Health as Foreign Policy, German-American Fulbright Commission and the American Council on Germany, Berlin, Germany, November 20–21, 2003); and Peter Grose, ed., *The Marshall Plan and its Legacy* (New York: Council on Floreign Relations, 1997.
5. Donald W. Roland, *History of the Office of the Coordinator of Inter-American Affairs: Historical Reports on War Administration* (Washington, D.C.: U.S. Government Printing Office, 1947).
6. Eugene T. Rossides, ed., *The Truman Doctrine of Aid to Greece: A Fifty-Year Retrospective* (Washington, D.C.: American Hellenic Institute Foundation, 1998).
7. Carol L. Graham, *Safety Nets, Politics, and the Poor: Transitions to Market Economies* (Washington, D.C., Brookings Institution, 1994), and Zsuzsa Ferge, "Social Policy Challenges and Dilemmas in Ex-Socialist Systems," in *Transforming Post-Communist Political Economies*, ed. Joan M. Nelson, Charles Tilly, and Lee Walker (Washington, D.C.: National Academy Press, 1997), 299.
8. Bruce W. Jentleson, ed., *Opportunities Missed, Opportunities Seized: Preventive Diplomacy in the Post-Cold War* World, Carnegie Commission On Preventing Deadly Conflict, New York: Carnegie Corporation of New York, Lanham, Maryland: Rowan & Littlefield Publishers, 1995, and Jordan S. Kassalow, *Why Health Is Important to U.S. Foreign Policy* (New York: Council on Foreign Relations, 2001.
9. Larry Diamond, *Promoting Democracy in the 1990s: Actors and Instruments, Issues and Imperatives. A Report to the Carnegie Commission on*

Preventing Deadly Conflict (New York: Carnegie Corporation of New York, December, 1995), and Patricio V. Marquez, *Dying Too Young: Addressing Premature Mortality and Ill Health Due to Non-Communicable Diseases and Injuries in the Russian Federation,* (Washington, D.C.: World Bank, 2005).
10. U.S. House of Representatives Speaker's Advisory Group on Russia, *Russia's Road to Corruption: How the Clinton Administration Exported Government Instead of Free Enterprise and Failed the Russian People*, 106th Cong., Washington, D.C., 2000.
11. Center for Strategic and International Studies, *CSIS Commission on Smart Power: A Smarter, More Secure America.* (Washington, D.C., Center for Strategic and International Studies, 2007).
12. National Institutes of Health, USA-Russia, *Twenty Years of Cooperation in Cardiopulmonary Research: 1972–1992* (Bethesda, Maryland: Office of International Programs, National Heart, Lung, and Blood Institute, 1994).
13. National Institutes of Health, U.S.-Russian Joint Symposium on New Developments in Cardiac Arrhythmias, Meridian International Center, Washington, D.C., May 23–25, 2001.
14. Thane Gustafson, *Wheel of Fortune: The Battle for Oil and Power in Russia*, (Cambridge, Massachusetts: Harvard University Press, 2012)
15. Peter Rutland, "Back to the Future: Economic Retrenchment in Russia," *Russian Analytical Digest* 180 (March 23, 2016).

About the Author

Edward J. Burger, Jr., MD., Sc.D., MACP

Dr. Edward Burger, Director, Eurasian Medical Education Program and President of the Institute for Health Policy Analysis, is responsible for the overall direction and support of the Eurasian Medical Education Program of the American College of Physicians in Russia. He holds a B.Sc. and an M.D. degree from McGill University and a Masters and Doctor of Science from Harvard. He served in the White House Office of the President's Science Advisor during the early 1970's. Dr. Burger helped develop cooperative programs in science, medicine and the environment with the Soviet Union during the period of detente. He served as leader of U.S. delegations to the Organization for Economic Cooperation and Development and served as Senior Scientific Advisor to the Economic Commission for Europe of the United Nations.

He was Professor of Community and Family Medicine at the Georgetown University Medical Center. In the 1960's, Dr. Burger was a Guggenheim Fellow and a member of the faculty of the Harvard School of Public and an Associate in the John F. Kennedy School of Government in Science and Public Policy. He is a member of a number of professional societies and is listed in Who's Who, Who's Who in America, Who's Who in Government, Who's Who in Health Care and in the American Men and Women in Science. Dr. Burger is the author of nearly 100 professional articles as well as several book-length works.

Index

Alaska, University of
American Russian Center 15
Alexander II, Emperor 1
All Union Commissariat of Health 3
American Bar Association 15
American Medical Association 13, 23
American College of Physicians 13,
 19, 23, 26-27, 30-32, 44, 69
American Diabetes Association 32
American International Health
 Alliance 9
Amur River 28, 42
Amur State Medical Academy 48
Antiballistic Missile Treaty 67

Baker, James 8
Bernstein, G. 32
Birobidzhan 21, 31
Bishovsky, V. 28
Blagoveschensk 35, 45, 47
Bolshevik Revolution 2

Cardiovascular Research Center 33
Cardiovascular disease 35-36, 52
Center for Strategic and
 International Security 66
Commission on Smart Power 66
Central and Eastern European Law
 Initiative (CEELI) 23
Cerebrovascular Disease 22

Chazov, E. 2, 32, 33
Chechnya 67
Chekov, A. 18, 47
Chugaev, Y. 27
Churin, I. 37
Cigarette smoking in Russia 35
Cochrane Collaboration 71
Commerce, U.S. Department of 20
Congressional Research Service 11

Daley, C. 39, 42
Demographic decline 5, 35-37
Denisov, I. 26, 29
Department for International
 Development (DFID) 10
Diabetes 22, 53
Dorovskih, V. 48
Dubna 51

Ekaterinburg 20, 27, 28, 31, 36,
 53-54
Envelope passing medicine 3
Eurasian Development Bank 10

Farmer, R. 12, 13
Fertility 5
Feshbach, M. 59
Field, M. 3
Fomine A. 28
Freedom Support Act 11

Gates, Bill and Melinda
 Foundation 22
Georgetown University 12, 45, 46
Georgia, Republic of 67
Global Fund for TB, Malaria and
 HIV/AIDS 44, 60
Greece, Point 4 Program 65

Hospital Partnership Program 9
Health Reform Project 9
Heifets, L 39-40
Herzen, A. 20
HIV/AIDS 22-23, 26, 35, 43-44,
 59-61

Institute for Inter-American Affairs
 64-65
International Monetary Fund 10
Irkutsk 35, 41, 45
Iseman, M. 32, 39-40

Japan 41
Jewish Autonomous region 21, 45
Johns Hopkins University 46

Kapitolino, N. 28
Kazan, 20, 21, 31-32, 36, 39, 54
Kazan State Medical Academy 21,
 29, 19
Kazan State Medical University 15,
 21, 29, 39, 71
Khabarovsk 15, 21, 27-28, 31, 36-37,
 45-46, 54
Khanti Mansisk 35
Khomenko, A., 39
Kogut, B. 28
Krasnov, V. 42

Leningrad Oblast 31, 35-36, 43, 45
Lexis-Nexis, Russia 33
Life Expectancy 3- 5

Marshall Plan 8, 10, 46
Medical Working Group 8, 9, 10
Melnikov, V. 30
Ministry of Foreign Affairs 70
Ministry of Health of the Russian
 Federation 19, 24-25, 27, 29, 30,
 31, 36, 49
Mortality in Russia
Mortality, premature 5
Moscow State Medical Academy
 25-26, 29-30
Mouzychenko, A. 33

National Institutes of Health
National Heart, Blood and
 Lung Institute; Cooperative
 Program on Cardiovascular and
 Pulmonary Disease 66
National Institute of Neurological
 Diseases and Stroke 17
National Jewish Medical and
 Research Center 32, 39
National Security Council 70
NATO 8, 67-68
New Jersey Medical Center 39
Nizhny Novgorod 20
Novosibirsk 33, 35, 41, 45
Novosibirsk TB Research
 Laboratory 41-42

Perlman, M. 39
Polyakova, T. 28
Portsmouth, Treaty of 18
Prison and tuberculosis 58-59

Reichman, L.39
Roosevelt, F.D. 65
Rockefeller Foundation 65
Rockefeller, Nelson 65
Rotary in Russia 33-34
Rotary International 33
Russian health insurance law19

Russian Academy of Medical
   Sciences 3, 68
Russian health insurance law 19
Russian Academy of Medical
   Sciences 3, 68

Sachs, J. 7
Sakha-Yakutia 15-16, 18, 35
Sakhalin Energy Corporation 34
Sakhalin Island 19
Shaimiev, Mintimer 21
Sirotin, A. 27, 37
Smolyak, V. 34
Soviet Academy of Medical
   Sciences 3
Soviet Academy of Sciences 3
State Research Center of Virology
   and Biotechnology (Vector)
   33-34
Stevens, T. 15
Strelkova, I. 28
Sverdlovsk 27, 37,39, 45-46
Sweet, D. 33, 44-45
Syrochkina, M. 27

Tatarstan 20-21, 36
Technical Aid to the
   Commonwealth of Independent
   States (TACIS) 10
Tuberculosis 10, 22, 54, 37-43, 55ff;
   BCG vaccine 38-39, 62; drug-
   resistant tuberculosis 39, 56;
   treatment methods in Russia 39,
   43; direct Observation Therapy
   Short Course (DOTS) 57
Tula 20, 3-31

Ukraine 43
UNAIDS 44
United Kingdom, Department
   for International Development
   (DIFID) 10

University of Alaska, American
   Russian Center 15
University of Kansas 44
University of Kentucky 29
University of Oregon 29
University of Rochester 27
University of Washington 29
Ural State Medical Academy 29
U.S. Agency for International
   Development 9, 23-24, 44, 70
U.S Centers for Disease Control
   and Prevention 59
U.S. Department of Commerce;
   Health Trade Mission to Russia
   20
U.S. Department of State 44, 70
U.S. National Intelligence Council 60
U.S. National Security Council 44
U.S. Senate, Foreign Operations
   Subcommittee of the Senate
   Appropriations Committee 23
U.S.-Soviet Cardiopulmonary
   Research Program 66

Vilius encephalitis 17
Vilius River 17
Virginia Mason Hospital 29
Vladivostok 21, 35

Walker, S. 32
Washington Coordinating
   Conference 8; Medical Working
   Group 8-9
White House 64-65; Office of the
   President's Science Adviser 12
World Bank 7, 10; Medical
   Equipment Project 10
World Health Organization 40-41, 56

Yakutsk 16, 45
Yastrebov, I. 27
Yellow fever 64

Yoshida, S. 33
Yuzhno Sakhalinsk 15, 18, 31, 33

Zemtsvo System 1-2
Ziganshina, L. 29

www.ingramcontent.com/pod-product-compliance
Lightning Source LLC
Chambersburg PA
CBHW031644170426
43195CB00035B/570